More praise for Sh

"The ALS Association is pleased to endorse ~~Share The C~~ [barcode obscures text] m-ple of a model of caring support that makes a meaningful difference for all who participate. The tools, techniques, and guidance in *Share The Care* offer a comprehensive plan that has provided valuable assistance to many people with ALS and their families."

—*Mary Lyon, R.N., M.N., vice president, patient services, the ALS Association*

"*Share The Care* transcends the pictures of what volunteerism is about. It is a step-by-step directive for creating a nurturing, heartfelt group of supportive partners in the caring process for an individual who is terminally ill, chronically ill, or disabled. It helps in maintaining their dignity and independence so they may live their lives more fully; the program is innovative, builds community, and is the wave of the future for caregiving."

—*Gail R. Mitchell, president, National Organization for Empowering Caregivers (NOFEC), www.nofec.org*

"A book for anyone who has ever wondered how to help a critically ill loved one and felt overwhelmed by their needs. *Share The Care* is clear, practical, and powerfully effective. What a blessing!"

—*Rachel Naomi Remen, M.D., author,* Kitchen Table Wisdom *and* My Grandfather's Blessings; *professor of clinical medicine, UCSF School of Medicine; founder and director, Institute for the Study of Health and Illness at Commonweal*

"It takes a village to care for patients dealing with cancer, both for those at diagnosis and for those with advanced disease. *Share The Care* is a superb model for activating and sustaining that village. The model enriches the lives of all involved."

—*James F. Cleary, M.D., associate professor of medicine (medical oncology), University of Wisconsin at Madison; director, Palliative Care Program, University of Wisconsin Comprehensive Cancer Center*

Share
The Care

How to Organize a Group to Care
for Someone Who Is Seriously Ill

Cappy Capossela
and Sheila Warnock

Revised and updated by Sheila Warnock

A FIRESIDE BOOK
Published by Simon & Schuster

New York   London   Toronto   Sydney

FIRESIDE
Rockefeller Center
1230 Avenue of the Americas
New York, NY 10020

Copyright © 1995, 2004 by Cappy Capossela and Sheila Warnock
All rights reserved,
including the right of reproduction
in whole or in part in any form.

This Fireside Edition 2004

FIRESIDE and colophon are registered trademarks of Simon & Schuster, Inc.

Designed by Ruth Lee Mui

For information regarding special discounts for bulk purchases,
please contact Simon & Schuster Special Sales at 1-800-456-6798
or business@simonandschuster.com

Manufactured in the United States of America

10   9   8   7   6   5   4

Library of Congress Cataloging-in-Publication Data

Capossela, Cappy.
    Share the care : how to organize a group to care for someone who is seriously ill /
Cappy Capossela and Sheila Warnock.—Rev. & updated by Sheila Warnock.
        p.   cm.
    Includes bibliographical references.
    1. Critically ill—Home care.   2. Critically ill—Social networks.   3. Caregivers.
4. Home nursing.   I. Warnock, Sheila.   II. Title.

RA 645.3.C36   2004
649.8—dc22   2004052757
ISBN: 978-0-7432-6268-2

This Book Is Dedicated

To Susan Farrow
who needed us

To Dr. Sukie Miller
who brought us together

and

To Susan's Funny Family
who went the distance

Joanne Ambrose
Eileen Brady
Barbara Delgado
Elissa Farrow Savos
Keri Farrow
Janet Frank
Jill Kirschen
Barbara Klein
Cheryl Howort Kramer
Eileen McClash
Pat Rogers
Ferne D. Ross
Myrna Schreibman
Sandy Tobin-Fishbein

and

To all the groups that followed
in their footsteps

Acknowledgments

Many people helped to make this book possible in their own unique and surprising ways. Susan's Funny Family was the first.

Special thanks to Susan's parents, Kay and Matthew Chmielewski; her ex-husband, Brian Farrow; her sister, Marion Giniger; her uncle, Sidney Wolf; and her friend David Gruber. They allowed us into their lives and supported us in helping.

Special thanks to Francine Cina for her courage and support. By asking us to create a Funny Family for her, she first made us see how the concept could help others.

Special thanks to all the other Funny Families who were open-minded and willing and who, in allowing us to help, made it possible to hone our existing systems and to create new ones.

Special thanks and acknowledgment to the people who supported us along the way, who with their unique and special talents were always ready when we needed them: Marc Bailin, Marc Blatte, Chris Corcoran, Dr. Dominick Masiello, Ken Nahoum, Bob Rabinowitz, and Barbara J. Zitwer.

Special thanks to our readers, Margot Dishner, Marc Kluender, Bonnie Lewis, and Sharon and Harvey Rosen, and to our typists, Lee Bodkin and Melanie Lee, who were also readers.

Special thanks to our own families, personal friends, and colleagues who have been rooting for us since day one.

It was difficult to translate our tears, fears, realizations, and systems into a book. Thanks to Susan Suffes of Warner Books, who first read our book proposal and encouraged us to go forward; to our agent, Lois De la

Haba, who believed it was a book; and to our astute and caring editor, Becky Cabaza, who turned it into a book.

Note: Many of the people who have been or still are part of Share The Care groups have contributed very personal thoughts, discoveries, insights, and experiences to this book. We thank them for this. Out of respect for their privacy, we have changed their initials in the quotes.

All names, addresses, and telephone numbers appearing on the forms are fictitious.

Additional Acknowledgments, 2004

The second edition of *Share The Care* would not be so rich without the wonderful contributions and incredible accomplishments of other groups. I thank all those who responded to my questions here in the United States and in Israel and Switzerland, in particular Amyee Balison, Marion Brandis, Cyndi Brzak, Ann Butterfield, Amrita Davidson, Brian Ewert, Kathryn Field, Maureen Gates, Mindy Gribble, Dorothea Joos, Melanie Lee, Susan Mayer-Zeitlin, Susan Mickel, Laura Shenkar, Frances Strayer, Barbara Walker, and Jennifer Wenzel. A warm thank-you for past contributions to Mary Stevens and her late husband, Rick, and Camille Massey. Also, thanks to Ann Ver Planck with the ALS Association in California for helping locate new groups.

A heartfelt thank-you to the members of Cappy's Brain Trust who gave me their personal feedback in my questionnaires, which served to document what we learned: Patty Abraham, Eileen Brady, Jim Capossela, Christina Churu, Kathy Mandry Cohn, Fran Heller, Lynda Klau, Margot Dishner Kluender, Steve Lance, Mary Manning, Richard Porter, Pat Rogers, and Elaine Sheresky, and to Anne Liebermann, who contributed verbal feedback. I am grateful to all the other members of the Brain Trust whose work pioneered new material for the book: Marc Bailin, Jean Blair, Mat Brady, Bob Christianson, Joan Cronin, Arthur English, Ron Gartner, Roger Hines, Jill Kirschen, Judy Kritzman, Dr. Dominick Masiello, Sharon Munsell, Dianne Stasi, Candice Vadala, Walter Van Green, and Ric Zuccarelli. A special thank-you to our support staff—Patsy Blackman, Oddett

Skeete, and Danielle Washington—for their everyday help. Included in my thanks are our very large team of free-floaters and those far away who lent their support, especially Seymour Carter, Dr. Sukie Miller, Jeffrey Nash, and Alexandria Thompson.

For her never-ending support and hard work, I would like to acknowledge Claire Culbertson, who followed up on groups in Wisconsin. A special thank-you to Marc Bailin for the ongoing gift of his expertise and to Patrick McNamara for his time and efforts. Thank you to Bob Stein and Tracy Landauer for their work with me on nonprofit matters.

A huge thanks to my wonderful readers—Bonnie Lewis, Dr. Sukie Miller, and Sharon Rosen—for their honest feedback when it was needed most.

My gratitude goes to Jay Stewart for gifting me with her editorial skills and comments. Because of her work with other Share The Care groups, her insights were incredibly valuable.

There would be no second edition if Trish Todd of Touchstone & Fireside Books had not recognized the value of what Share The Care was accomplishing. A warm thank-you to my editors, Christina Duffy and Sara Schapiro, for guiding me through the process of getting the updated *Share The Care* ready for press.

I would also like to warmly acknowledge the members of the board of directors of sharethecaregiving, Inc., and all my other personal friends, family, and colleagues for cheering me on. Last but not least, a special thank-you (with love) to Cappy's mom, Josephine Capossela.

Contents

PART 4

Keeping the Group (and Yourself) Going

PART 5

Beyond the Group: Changed Lives

Introduction

Share The Care was released in December 1995. In January 1996 the *Washington Post* printed an excellent article entitled "Friends in Deed," * detailing the concept of group caregiving and our story. In April, I was sent a clipping from the same paper, entitled *"Friends in Deed, II."* It was about a woman who, inspired by the first article, started a group for her friend who was dying of lymphoma. Although the friend died within a few months, her group vowed to continue their support for her husband and seven-year-old daughter through the rest of the year. This included a fund-raiser (the subject of the article) to pay for the overwhelming medical expenses that had accumulated. When Cappy and I read the article we were moved to tears. It was our first proof that *Share The Care* was making a difference.

Over the years, we occasionally heard from groups and individuals who took time to thank us for writing the book. Through newspaper articles, letters, phone calls, and e-mails we were able to document that *Share The Care* was being used in at least thirty-three states (and later, other parts of the world). It became a highly respected manual in the field of caregiving as groups came together to help people suffering from diseases and the elderly in need of assistance. The media interviewed us about our experiences in "Susan's Funny Family." We gave lectures to health-care professionals and social services students about our new approach to caregiving. We were honored with an invitation to contribute a short piece, "How to Share the Care," to the PBS Web site for On Our Own Terms: Moyers on

* "Friends in Deed (A Special Family)," by Barbara Mathias, *Washington Post*, January 2, 1996; and "Update: Friends in Deed, II," *Washington Post*, April 9, 1996.

Dying.* Then we learned the University of Wisconsin Comprehensive Cancer Center had secured several grants from the Susan G. Komen Breast Cancer Foundation to fund the use of the Share The Care model to help women with breast cancer. They even produced a video about an actual group for a woman named Michelle.

In January 2002, the unthinkable happened. My dear friend and co-author, Cappy, was diagnosed with a malignant brain tumor. I raced to put together a Share The Care group to help her through an indescribably difficult illness. We lost her ten months later. Sometime during this experience, I made a major life decision. Fueled by my third experience as a primary caregiver, armed with the support of friends, family, and Cappy's group, and confident with the inner knowledge that all my life experiences had been prepping me for this, I founded a nonprofit organization. Its mission is to promote group caregiving using the Share The Care model as a proven option for caregivers everywhere.

In April of 2003 Share The Care gave birth to sharethecaregiving, Inc. A Web site for the model, http://www.sharethecare.org, went up in August, and by December 1 we had filed an application for exemption with the IRS and registered with the New York State Charities Bureau. You can read about sharethecaregiving, its mission, and more in chapter 31, or check the Web site for the most current information.

In late 2003, I got the green light not only to update *Share The Care* in terms of technology and resources but also to include new hands-on ideas pioneered by Cappy's group and other real-life groups who have generously contributed their information for this new edition.

One of my dreams for sharethecaregiving came to life today. For the first time, I was able to connect a group (no longer functioning) with another (less than a year old) for support and ideas. One has been down the road of caring for a loved one with ALS while the other is struggling with how to cope as their friend's ALS progresses at a rapid pace. They are in different states, but through their e-mails I could see a fit: a willingness to help and the openness to receive. It was gratifying to help them find each other.

Working on the new edition of *Share The Care* these past few months

* "How to Share the Care" by Cappy Capossella and Sheila Warnock, http://www.thirteen.org/onourownterms/articles/share.html.

has been paving the road for my work with sharethecaregiving. We're getting the road signs up as we speak: Collaborate, Teach, Compassion, Support, and Share, to name a few. These are the guideposts that are going to move and connect us in ways we haven't even dreamed of.

Sheila Warnock

February 2004

Foreword to the 1995 Edition

We live and prosper, sicken and die, too much alone. Families get smaller; spouses separate, move, and change careers—we all know how it is.

Paradoxically, we also live too much in immense systems of strangers who serve and are served by us: schools, businesses, highways, malls, clinics, and hospitals. These human but nonpersonal systems are efficient, but they cannot supply us with intimate attention, love, tenderness, and understanding.

The psychotherapist works within this paradox of solitude and system as well. Our aloneness is punctuated by intense periods of time shared with regular patients. On the other hand, there are the impersonal systems of peer review boards, insurance companies, and patient referrals to other professionals in other bureaucracies.

A few years ago, I was especially moved by a patient named Susan who was stricken with a relentless cancer. In the course of her illness, Susan—whose case runs through the pages of this book—met intimately with me for a few hours a week while she was otherwise perpetually engaged with the health-care system and its subsystems of hospitals, private practitioners, clinical laboratories, and drugstores.

In the course of our time together, I learned, almost in passing, that though she lived alone, Susan had a large number of friends and acquaintances scattered nearby. Nevertheless, when she needed the kind of daily, ongoing, deep personal attention that bureaucracies cannot give and geographically dispersed family cannot provide, she seemed to both of us starkly alone. Her friends came into her daily life only for brief moments—to meet for lunch, to accompany her to a doctor's appointment, to phone in a late-night call of comfort and support. She was stranded. Society has sophisticated physical apparatuses to keep us alive as long as possible, but not much to offer us for dealing with the solitude, fear, guilt, fatigue, and other trials that accompany severe illness.

Susan needed, as so many of us will, an old-fashioned, on-site, extended family, an ideal one that would not burn out in the long process of abiding with the severely ill. Feeling for her suffering, foreseeing her slow dying, I suggested she gather together her friends and acquaintances—people who, for the most part, did not know one another—and that they form such a "family." I organized the first meeting and helped with two later gatherings. The splendid group—Susan's Funny Family, as they came to be known—did all the rest, and in great detail, as the reader will see.

The small group can work miracles, as our common experience shows us. We know this even from the creaky, lurching successes of the bureaucracies that characterize most of our public institutions, from business to politics. We know it also when warfare calls on us for great sacrifices and ordinary men and women in combat do heroic deeds. Soldiers are impelled not by abstract notions of flag and country, according to postwar researchers, but by loyalty and involvement in the group, the platoon that keeps every army functioning in the face of death. The family group is another such potent conformation, and so are the historic, primitive healing groups assembled by tribal healers to cast out spells, to cure psychosis, to bring a glimpse of the divine through ritual.

In this book, the brave people who created Susan's Funny Family share their knowledge and experience with those of you who want to join together to form a caregiving group for someone suffering from illness, injury, or disability, short-term or long-term.

The benefits are enormous. Not only does the patient get higher quality and more comprehensive care in every sense—from physical to emotional well-being—but the caregivers themselves are supported, healed, and even ennobled.

Sometimes we need to stop living so much alone. This extraordinary book shows a way.

Sukie Miller, Ph.D.
Penngrove, California

PART 1

What's a Caregiver Group and Who Needs One?

CHAPTER ONE

How This Book Came to Be Written

Cappy's Story

I met Susan Farrow when we shared a summerhouse on Fire Island, a narrow strip of beach that runs parallel to Long Island. Susan was four feet eleven inches of sass, a fiery redhead with a sharp wit and a sexy demeanor, a demanding job, and two children who were living with her after her divorce.

There were eight of us in that summerhouse, and when I think back on those carefree Fire Island days, the two things I remember most about Susan were her fierce commitment to having fun and our long conversations about men. We shared a passion for life and a love of passion. We were in our mid-thirties then.

But we were also ambitious women, and as our careers heated up we began to lose touch. I was an advertising copywriter (writing screenplays and songs on the side). She was the head of the promotion department of Lever Brothers (raising two children on the side).

I first heard she had cancer from Sheila, who was one of my oldest and best friends. I remember being shocked that Susan, of all people, could have such a serious disease, but when I tried to talk to Susan about it, she said there was nothing to worry about, that they "got it all." Although she had had several surgeries and radiation treatments, she treated it as an unpleasant, temporary interruption of her life, and I was happy to treat the news of it pretty much the same way.

On the rare occasions I did see her (usually as part of a four-woman birthday group who celebrated birthdays four times a year), we talked about our careers, men, clothes, movies, New York, politics, anything but cancer, which she called "the Big C."

I didn't know it at the time, but Susan had a rare form of cancer that had started in the salivary gland and had metastasized to the bones. The tumors were slow growing at first, so there were long periods of time when she could tell herself it was gone and was never coming back. Then another tumor would appear on another bone and she would be back in the hospital or under the radiation machine.

Through it all, for years, she worked (and even managed to get a promotion), took care of her kids, and continued an on-again, off-again love relationship. She refused to join cancer support groups and never admitted the seriousness of her disease to anyone (I suspect not even to herself). I was content to be in denial with her, since I had never wrapped my mind around the concept of death and had never been sick a day in my life. In those days, I was a blur of activity, totally and relentlessly unaware of limitations. As Susan was fond of saying, I was one of those people to whom nothing bad had ever happened. I still had both my parents. I looked much younger than my age and had boundless energy and a Peter Pan optimism. Not only had I never had children, I'd never had to take responsibility for another living creature, not even a pet.

Then on March 15, 1988, I got the phone call that would change my life. Susan, who by this time had been struggling with cancer for four and a half years, told me through her tears that she could no longer take care of herself alone. She was exhausted, terrified, almost hysterical as she asked me if I would come to a meeting at Dr. Sukie Miller's office. Dr. Miller was her psychotherapist and had urged her to invite her friends to a meeting to see if, together, we could find a way to help her. Dr. Miller, who had been actively involved in health-care issues for many years (and who had been an early advocate of group work), was uniquely qualified to conduct the meeting that would turn a gathering of ordinary people into a powerful caregiver group.

Susan invited eighteen of her friends to the meeting; twelve of us came. We were given very short notice to attend and I was frazzled. I had just left a job as advertising copywriter to open my own music company and was flying to Los Angeles for a recording session the morning after the meeting.

I knew only a few people in the room, and Sheila was my only really close friend there.

I was shocked as my feisty friend Susan broke down and told us her medical horror story, how she had eight doctors, none of whom talked to each other, how she was afraid she might have to quit her job, how she had to have a test immediately because if a tumor was growing on her spine, she could be paralyzed. She was angry, almost hysterical, and convinced that no one in the room could help her.

Dr. Miller had a four-foot-tall dollhouse in her office, exquisitely furnished, and I remember wishing I could crawl into it and stay there until the meeting was over. Dr. Miller went around the room and asked us each for one word describing our feelings. Mine was *terror*. I had never been very comfortable in groups, and this one was especially difficult because I was convinced everyone could see how scared I was.

Three hours passed in a blur, as we shared feelings and did exercises designed to help us come together as a group. We shared our strengths and weaknesses, formed teams, and answered strange questions, such as what did each of us think we would get from being in the group. When it was over, I flew out the door, glad to have the excuse of an early morning flight. I had agreed to be part of the group, but I wasn't sure I'd be able to come through.

As I write this, that was five years ago. The group that came to Dr. Miller's office that evening stayed together and took almost total care of Susan until she died three and a half years later. Only one person dropped out; others were added. As we went along, we developed a unique system for caring for someone seriously ill. We became known as Susan's Funny Family.

In those three and a half years, I learned a lot about sickness and dying, but that was nothing compared to what I learned about living. I learned what it was to put yourself in someone else's place. I learned how to stop doing and just be. I learned that by accepting limitations you make life a richer, deeper experience. I learned people can be healed even if they are not cured.

Mostly, I learned about the special power of a group, and I found bonds of friendship and love that are more powerful than disease and stronger than fear. I am not the person I was five years ago. Today, I lead Funny Family caregiver groups with my best friend and coauthor, Sheila Warnock, and it is still a mystery to me that I am now a source of strength for other people who feel as frightened and inadequate as caregivers as I once did.

Sheila's Story

One of the few things Susan and I had in common was our red hair. Otherwise, we were a real contrast in personalities. She was outgoing, gutsy, and very much of the world. I was laid-back, creative, and into exploring the more mystical side of life. We shared group summerhouses and hung out in the city, going to movies, parties, and street fairs. As an artist, I loved helping her daughters, Keri and Elissa, with their costumes and makeup on Halloween, and Susan loved giving me advice on any subject whether I wanted it or not. Yet we enjoyed each other's perspectives and were the best of friends.

But unlike her other friends, I knew of her war with cancer right from the beginning. One night I was at her apartment when she fretted over the lump that had appeared out of nowhere on the side of her head, just over the ear. "It's probably a cyst, but go get it checked out right away," I remember saying to her. Then her doctor sent her to a specialist who ordered surgery to remove it immediately.

I took her to the hospital, stayed with her kids, and visited her minutes after they brought her back from the recovery room, her face still stained yellow from the antiseptic. I'll never forget when the surgeon came to speak with Susan and asked me to leave the room (because I wasn't family). I felt sad, awkward, and angry all at the same time. I thought, Why couldn't I be there for my friend? She was all alone except for the stranger in the next bed when the doctor told her, "It was malignant, but I think I got it all."

During her recuperation she told me that she had decided to keep her cancer a secret. I listened and groped for words as she agonized that the operation had left her, for the time being, with an ugly, distorted smile. It all felt so unreal. Susan had always looked healthy and attractive, and she was my peer. How could all this be happening?

Over the next four years, I did my best to help her in emotional and practical ways as the cancer came and receded like the ocean. There were many more surgeries, radiation treatments, and tests.

But this was only half of my caregiving story. At the same time that Susan was fighting her cancer, my mother, who lived several hours away, was just beginning what was to be a long and painful decline. My father had died a couple of years prior, and my brother and sister-in-law lived out of the country. I suddenly found myself her sole caregiver.

Over time, I learned, by absolute necessity, an astounding number of things: how to buy and sell a home, drive a car, deal with emergencies, manage doctors, and navigate the intricacies of Medicare and Medicaid. Eventually I had to find a nursing home for my mother because she could no longer walk or be alone and I couldn't make a living and care for her at the same time.

I called on strengths within myself I didn't even know existed and did everything I could for both Susan and my mother. There was only one very important person I overlooked . . . myself. My life had just stopped. I rarely saw any of my other friends, never dated, and became obsessed with worry. It didn't occur to me to ask for help even though I was always on the brink of tears and couldn't sleep. My personal aspirations to pursue an acting career were shoved to the back burner, and even my work as a freelance art director in advertising (which was paying most of the bills) was suffering because I never had time to find new clients or be available when the ones I had needed me. I was always on my way out to solve another crisis.

Then Susan told me she had to have yet another complicated test, a test that required hospitalization. This time she was really on the verge of a breakdown, and at the insistence of her therapist, Dr. Miller, she agreed to call a group of friends together to ask for help. She knew I was totally burnt out and she was terrified of doing battle with no help at all.

The night the Funny Family was born, I looked at the sea of faces in the room and all I remember was feeling a huge wave of relief. I wasn't quite sure how this group could possibly work. I wasn't very big on groups and had only very recently joined a women's support group just to air some of the overwhelming feelings I was having. In that group I had just begun to sense the possibilities of sharing.

Being part of Susan's group was the most important caregiving lesson I could ever learn: how to take care of myself while I took care of others. As I learned to share workloads, decisions, feelings, and responsibilities—to ask for help when I needed it and allow myself to say no sometimes—my life began to return to me.

In one night, with the encouragement of Dr. Miller, this group of strangers pooled their heads, hearts, experience, and compassion and went to work. It is amazing to me how much I personally gained from that experience and the astounding difference the group made in the quality of my life. I learned so much from them, found more courage within myself because of them, and was able to express my frustrations, anger, and fear to them and know that they understood completely. To this day, we are bonded together by the three and a half years of tears and laughter we shared while helping Susan.

I never dreamed that I would be sharing my experience and writing a book on this subject with my friend Cappy. I feel privileged to be doing this work and to be one of the midwives at the births of so many new caregiver groups.

The First Funny Family

Over the course of the three and a half years that Susan's Funny Family was together, we were astounded at the power of a group of ordinary people. We cooked and cleaned, shopped and visited, accompanied Susan to doctors, radiation appointments, hospitals, seminars. One of us did her insurance forms and paperwork while another coordinated her doctors, X-rays, and tests.

One member wrote a screenplay with Susan about their experiences with the group. Another member totally organized Susan's daughter's wedding, when Susan was unable to lift a telephone. Two of us and Susan's older daughter, Keri, took Susan to the Bahamas for an alternative treatment, and over the course of six months, several members each spent one or two weeks with her in the Bahamas because she couldn't be alone.

We baked her kiwi tarts, painted her toenails, held her when she was in pain, laughed with her when it was a good day. Eventually, we washed her hair and put on her makeup, wrote out her checks and arranged for in-home health care when she could no longer leave her bed. We learned about her medications, gave her injections, and finally arranged for the help of hospice for her last days.

We amazed Susan and we surprised ourselves. But the miraculous part is that if you talk to the individual members, no one regrets having been part of the group and no one would say it was too much. In helping Susan, we helped each other. Through crises, through making important decisions together, we held each other's hands, discovered the enormous healing power of a group, and formed a bond so deep we believed it could see us through anything.

After Susan's death, we knew that no one person (or even two or three) could or should have to cope alone with what it had taken twelve of us to do. We became determined to share with others what we had learned. Our chance came sooner than we thought.

Another Group Is Formed

Susan died on September 14, 1991. Six months later, we got a phone call from a friend of Susan's named Francine, who had been suffering from non-Hodgkin's lymphoma for many years. She had met Susan at Cancer Care, a support group for patients, and they stayed in touch while Francine's cancer went into remission and Susan's grew worse. Susan often spoke of her Funny Family to Francine. After Susan died, Francine's cancer reappeared and she was told she needed to have several courses of chemotherapy followed by a bone-marrow transplant, a procedure that would leave her in a weak and vulnerable state for most of a year. Her aging parents and her sixteen-year-old daughter had been her only caregivers, and she was worried that coping with this dangerous and difficult treatment would be too much for them.

Francine described what she was about to go through, explained that she had a lot of friends who were trying to help but didn't know how, and then in a timid voice asked if we thought she might need a Funny Family.

Our first reaction was to say "Great." Our second was "Maybe Dr. Miller can lead it." But Francine wasn't in therapy and neither were most of her friends, and she wasn't comfortable with that idea. She wanted us to lead the meeting. The prospect of leading the meeting without Dr. Miller was daunting. Even though Cappy and I both had been in hundreds of business meetings, this was different. This involved people's lives. We knew that if we did it well, we could actually help change the course of the next year for Francine and her friends.

We went to see Dr. Miller and told her we didn't know if we could do this meeting without her. She said that indeed we could—and even do it better than she because we had lived through it. She instructed us to gather the members of Susan's group and Francine and her friends and simply do a set of sharing exercises. We would share who we were and how we had come to know Susan; they would share who they were and how they knew Francine. We would share what we got out of being in Susan's group; they would share what they hoped to get out of being in Francine's group. We would not position ourselves as experts but merely give them the information, systems, and forms we had developed while taking care of Susan. We did not have to have all the answers, she said. All we had to do was share from the heart and keep the meeting on track.

We asked Francine to make a list of her friends and acquaintances who might want to help, and then sat down and tried to remember what had been the most important things in our meeting with Dr. Miller and what had made a difference. In preparing for the meeting, we were surprised at the wealth of experience and information we had to pass on.

We consulted with Dr. Miller, planned the evening carefully, and divided it into two parts. In part one we would do the exercises we had done with Dr. Miller, and in part two we would pass along the practical worksheets we had developed.

When we called the members of Susan's group, having not spoken to many of them for months, we were immediately a family again. All twelve original members wanted to participate. Francine called to say fourteen of her friends were coming. On the night of the meeting, we had exercises to do and forms to give out. We had sandwiches, soft drinks, and cookies to serve during a break. We had name tags for everyone.

The room was filled with concern, discomfort, fear, and confusion, as well as love and an intense desire to help. Francine was very nervous. Her friends were apprehensive. We were apprehensive. But the minute we began to share who we were and what we had done, the atmosphere in the room changed. We shared our experiences and memories, and realized that along with the difficulties and the pain, there had also been laughter, profound insights, and miracles.

As Francine's friends talked, it was very moving to see how much they cared for her, how much they wanted to help. There was warmth, laughter, and many tears as Francine talked about her illness, what she needed, and how difficult it was for her to ask for help. We passed out the forms we had developed and explained the systems we had inaugurated. We watched in amazement as her friends began to see what was needed, to move themselves into commitment, to plan the practical steps they needed to take, and to bond together as a group.

We will never forget the special power of that evening as a group of well-meaning but frightened, unsure people became Francine's Funny Family right before our eyes! Here are some of the things her friends had to say:

> I felt many things at that meeting. Sadness about Francine's illness, the realization of what could happen in the future, pride in seeing my "sisters" giving unconditionally, and the feeling that Francine felt privileged and felt our love. (L.N.)

> It was an incredible experience and I felt very lucky to be there. It was all I could talk about for weeks. (K.T.)

> It felt very spiritual because of all the love in the room. I have never felt anything like that before. I remember thinking that Francine has given us such a gift of sharing and how lucky I was to be chosen. (B.B.)

> I recall the organization and effort that went into the meeting. The dedication and commitment of Susan's Funny Family. The fact that Susan had no relatives nearby. How collectively everyone was able to assist Susan and the honesty and nondenial of Susan's disease. (C.R.)

The next morning, Cappy and I realized that something unique had happened. We had found a way to share the burden of coping with serious illness, a way to take care of the caregiver. We realized how helpful it would have been if everything we had learned had been written down, and we resolved to document our caregiving system in a book. As we began to work on it, we realized we were uniquely suited to the task. One of us had never been a caregiver and had been scared to death, and the other had nearly burnt out being a caregiver. Between us, we covered the two categories of caregivers struggling with serious illnesses today.

Since that first meeting we have started many other caregiver groups, refining the meeting but basically following the same format. Each time, no matter who is in the group, no matter how much fear or resistance there is, no matter whether the person has been sick for a long time or has just found out about the illness, we have been moved by the goodness of people, by the deep desire to help and the longing to be part of something meaningful.

This Book Is for You If . . .

- You've never been a caregiver and someone with a serious, complex, demanding illness turns to you for help. You love them, want to be there for them, but are afraid.
- You're already taking care of someone who is ill and your own life is beginning to fall apart; you're tired and burnt out and there doesn't seem to be anyone else to help.

Now you don't have to do it all alone. No matter how scared you are, no matter how sick they are, whether you've ever been a "joiner" or led a meeting, with the help of this book you can create a group to share the care. You can make caregiving a healing, meaningful, and less stressful experience for everyone. You can take total care of the person you love—and take care of yourself too.

CHAPTER TWO

Do You Need a Caregiver Group?

You Just Found Out

You've just found out your wife (husband, best friend, daughter, mother, father, son, significant other) has been diagnosed with a life-threatening illness (cancer, AIDS, Alzheimer's) or has had an accident or sudden health crisis (heart attack, stroke). They can't believe it's happening to them—and neither can you.

They're shocked, fearful, angry, upset, and overwhelmed—and so are you. You stare at them helplessly, trying to see the cancer, but they look fine. Maybe they've never been sick a day in their lives and are sure the doctor made a mistake.

They have to have surgery (radiation, bone scans, MRIs, X-rays, bypasses, transplants). They have to make difficult, complicated decisions quickly.

She's your best friend and you both live alone on opposite sides of a big city. You both have high-powered, demanding jobs. She was in a serious car accident over the weekend and will need extensive help while recovering from several broken bones. They call you from the hospital.

He's your neighbor. You both live in a small rural community sixty miles from the nearest hospital. He was diagnosed with cancer and will need radiation treatments at that hospital every day for the next four weeks. His wife died last year. He asks if you can take him to his treatments.

She's your youngest child and you've just been told she has leukemia. You're the mother of three, separated from your husband, and working a part-time job. Your daughter will require your total attention.

She's your mother and she lives with your aunt in Florida. She has been suffering from Alzheimer's but now it's becoming impossible for one person to care for her. Your aunt calls you. You live in California with your husband and two children.

He's your father-in-law and he lives with you and your wife. He suffers a major stroke that leaves him partially paralyzed. Your business requires you to travel constantly and money is tight. Your wife is pregnant with your first child.

He's your fiancé and he's just been diagnosed with AIDS. You were planning to be married next July. You feel as if your life just fell apart.

They Turn to You

Someone who's never shown emotion suddenly starts to cry in your arms. Someone who's always been quiet and soft-spoken begins to scream at a doctor while you're with him. They want your help but they don't know how to ask for it, they don't want to ask for it, they've never asked for it, or they are afraid you won't come through.

You're thrown into a whole new world filled with strange procedures and frightening words . . . biopsies, MRIs, metastasize, T-cells, bypass, bone marrow. They ask you to talk to doctors you've never heard of . . . oncologists, radiologists, orthopedic surgeons, neurologists. They ask for your advice on life-and-death matters. Should they get a second opinion? A third? Should they have radiation or chemotherapy? They ask you to break the news to a husband or wife or mother or child.

You suddenly realize you've never taken care of someone with a serious illness and you don't know how.

You don't know what to say to them or what to expect. Maybe the only person you ever knew who died was your grandmother. Maybe you're afraid of hospitals, intimidated by doctors. Or maybe you have a very hectic life as it is and know you don't have the time to take care of someone. Maybe you just started your own business and you work from eight in the morning till nine at night. Maybe you've got three kids of your own or you just started graduate school.

You feel helpless. Feelings that have been buried for years begin to surface. Life takes on a new heaviness. Suddenly it occurs to you that if this could happen to them it could happen to you, and you want to run away. You find yourself thinking about your own mortality, crying for no reason, wondering if there is a God, hugging your children fiercely, obsessed with keeping busy. You realize you never told this person you love him or her out loud. You have an anxiety attack in the middle of *General Hospital.* You can't get out of bed in the morning.

You Start to Do It All Alone

You cope the best you can. After all, it's your sister, your mom, your friend, your fiancée, and you want to be a good daughter, friend, lover, husband. You tell yourself it's only until they get better. It can't be tougher than your job, your husband's moods, raising three kids. Doctors and nurses do it all the time. But you discover it's more demanding than you think.

Taking care of someone you love is different from taking care of someone as a health professional. Not only do you have to stretch your own life in a hundred different ways, but you're also losing the support of someone who was once there for you. Not only are you confronting someone else's fears about pain, death, and dying, but you are confronting your own.

You're exhausted after taking them to the doctor. They want to tell you every grim detail and you don't want to hear it. You find yourself going blank when a radiologist is talking to you. You don't seem to be able to set limits on how much time you'll spend on their health problems.

Your emotional swings are as manic as theirs.

One minute you hate them and the next you feel closer to them than ever before. On the one hand, you resent them for taking so much out of you and on the other you feel good about being so needed, honored to be doing something so meaningful.

You Become the Main Caregiver

The illness drags on. You run from work to the hospital. Chronically sleep-deprived, you snap at your own family, forget to pick up the dog, lose your car keys. You feel totally responsible, guilty, embarrassed at your own fears and your inability to talk about them, or even to tell the sick person how much you love him or her.

Sick people are not the people they've always been. Their mood swings are frightening. They're angry at you for no reason. They're demanding, cranky, hostile. Nothing you do is right. You're angry at them but you feel too guilty to say anything.

You even feel guilty for being healthy.

You begin to neglect your own health. You stop going to the health club. Your job begins to suffer. You haven't told the people in the office what's going on, so they don't understand why you're not yourself. You may not even realize you're different.

You begin to withdraw socially, never having the energy or down time for fun. Your sex drive seems to shrivel up. You never laugh anymore. You may begin to lose your own friends. You certainly don't have time for their problems—which, next to the ones your sick friend has, are nothing. Week after week, you find yourself canceling that class or tennis match or movie.

Your own friends or family or lover or co-workers won't know what you're going through unless they've been caregivers themselves, so it may seem that you're always complaining, always tired, no longer any fun. They may even think you have a drug problem or a drinking problem. You may begin to feel a great loneliness.

Why don't you ask for help?

Whom would you ask? Who wants to hear about sickness? We live in a youth-obsessed, production-driven, materialistic society that has only just begun to accept death and dying as a fact of life, let alone as a mystery to be respected and revered.

No one wants to confront illness unless forced to. So if you ask for help, you run the risk of turning off your own friends. Even if help is there, you may not see it. You may be creating an invisible wall around yourself.

So you keep going. The problems mount. They need another operation. The nursing home still doesn't have a bed. They want to talk about death and you don't. The insurance company won't pay for live-in help. They ask if they can move in with you. Just when you need your objectivity, strength, and clearheadedness the most, you feel spacey, disconnected, confused. If things continue this way, you feel like you're going to fall apart. A "burnt-out" caregiver put it this way:

> When trying to take care of someone by yourself, you begin to feel like you're in a dark, murky whirlpool with no escape. You can't even begin to imagine there could be a way out of the never-ending problems, setbacks, and depressing feelings. (S.S.)

Share The Care

If you've been asked to care for someone who is seriously ill and you don't know how or are afraid, or if you've already become a full-time caregiver and you're beginning to burn out, you can get more help than you ever dreamed possible.

You can put together a group of people to share the care of your loved one. In fact, you can create a caregiver family from friends and acquaintances that people will want to be part of, a "family" that will nurture not only the person who is ill but everyone who is a part of it.

At first putting together a caregiver group may seem impossible. Perhaps you've already tried to get people to help and discovered they were too busy or they made promises and didn't come through. Perhaps they helped out for a while but then dropped out. Maybe they've told you that doctors and hospitals frighten them or they have too many problems of their own. Maybe a good friend has distanced herself after hearing about your husband's illness, or a daughter has stopped calling. Maybe you're convinced that *your* friends, *your* neighbors, *your* co-workers, *your* relatives aren't the kind of people who want to get involved.

It's true that many people have formed support groups that haven't really worked, or they've worked for a while and then fallen apart. The difference is that the Share The Care approach does not result in just a support group. It's the basis for a powerful group system that provides every practical tool you need, a system that has been refined through the experiences of many groups.

The Share The Care system begins with a meeting where several group exercises and practical worksheets help to set everyone on the same road and create both a lasting emotional bonding and a strong group organization. It gives you something to fall back on when things get difficult, a ground of being that keeps the group going, keeps the individual members from burning out, and keeps the group together. So when you begin to form your group, don't be put off if at first people seem reluctant.

It is natural for *individuals* to run from illness. People often fear calling a person who is ill and offering help. They're afraid they'll have to do something they can't stand or aren't good at. They're afraid they'll end up being the only one to help. They're afraid of being used, afraid that people will see their weaknesses, that their husbands or wives won't support them. They're already doing too much and are afraid to add to their already overburdened lives. So they put off calling and feel terribly guilty while their sick friend concludes they just don't care about them anymore. But a *group* approach is different.

People Want to Help

In spite of how scary illness is, people do want to make a difference, to contribute. According to the Bureau of Labor Statistics of the U.S. Department of Labor, "Both the number of volunteers and the volunteer rate rose over the year ended in September 2003." The BLS notes that "about 63.8 million people did volunteer work at some point from September 2002 to September 2003, up from 59.8 million for a similar period ended in September 2002. The volunteer rate grew to 28.8 percent, up from 27.4 percent." *

In his inspiring book *Heroes After Hours,* David C. Forward chronicles hundreds of extraordinary acts of employee volunteerism and talks about why people volunteer:

> I really enjoy the camaraderie of working on projects alongside my co-workers, but there's more: the thrill that I get when the AIDS baby I'm feeding gives me an ear-to-ear smile; the warmth that permeates my

* U.S. Department of Labor, "Volunteering in the United States, 2003," http://www.bls.gov/news.release/volun.nr0.htm

whole body when the lonely senior citizen takes my hand after I stop to chat with her during my Meals on Wheels route; the hug I got from my at-risk mentoring student as he beamed with pride after getting the first A in his life. These are the real reasons people volunteer. And the numbers are increasing, because once you have experienced it, you can never ignore a plea for help again.

Volunteerism seems to be bringing great meaning into modern life and seems to be able to heal the wounds caused by isolation. Yet if so many Americans are volunteering to help charities, hospitals, and nonprofit organizations, why are so many individual caregivers taking care of their loved ones alone? Perhaps it's because it's too close to home. People are afraid to intrude. They don't know what's enough, what's too much. They don't know what the sick person needs or wants because the sick person has never asked. Often, there are many people who want to help but they are all duplicating each other's efforts. Perhaps it is simply that they don't know what to do.

But give them a specific task or a job they're suited for and they will lose their fear. A simple "Aunt Jane, you make such a wonderful chicken casserole—maybe you would bake one for Joe and deliver it for his dinner on Thursday?" can make two people very happy. Give them a group to work with and a structure to fit into, and they will feel less anxious. Give them an opening to say yes or no and they may come back with a different or even a better offer. "I can't help with doing errands for Mary this week but I'd be happy to help out next week, and I have a great video I think she'd enjoy." Give them a safe, proven system to follow, a caregiver family to belong to, and a group to share it all with, and you will see that there are more than enough people to help.

You Don't Have to Be a Professional

You don't have to be a therapist, nurse, or specialist to do this. It requires no professional training, but it uses all the skills you already have. It doesn't cost anything, yet it could save weeks, months, even years of your life.

When Dr. Miller first asked Susan to invite her friends to a meeting,

Susan said there were only one or two people who would come. But Dr. Miller persisted until finally Susan came up with eighteen names. Twelve of us came. We were from different pockets of Susan's life—from her office, from PTA meetings, from the summerhouse we shared. Some of us were her old friends, some casual acquaintances. Most of us were complete strangers to each other.

We were in our thirties, forties, and fifties. We were single, married, gay, straight, divorced, with children and without, one of us a grandmother. We had a wide variety of occupations. Some of us were highly successful, others struggling and unemployed. Among the people who came to the meeting were an actress, an advertising executive, a housewife, a hairdresser, a corporate executive, and a secretary.

We lived as close as upstairs and as far away as the next state. Later, the group expanded to include Susan's cousin, a sister of one of the members (who was a nurse), a voice teacher, and a jazz pianist.

Although we were a competent, intelligent group, none of us had ever dealt with a terminally ill person for any extended period, none of us had any special training (except the nurse, who said being in the group gave her a whole new perspective on caregiving), and none of us had ever coped with the dying and death of a young woman who was a friend.

When we started, we knew very little about disease, doctors, and hospitals, and nothing of the intense needs of chronically ill people. But we stayed together for three and a half years. During that time, several members were added to the group, only one person dropped out, and no one experienced burnout.

Listen to some of the people who were apprehensive about being in a caregiver family and did it anyway:

I just had such a need to do *something* for Lois. Whatever that was going to be, I had no idea. I needed to be a part of her life and to help her in any way possible. I also wanted a better understanding of what she was to go through so that it could possibly alleviate some of my own terror concerning cancer. She was so strong—I needed to witness her strength. After being a part of her [group], I realized how strong she was but also how strong I could be. I learned about *choosing life* from her and the trials an individual's body must sometimes endure. My own priorities in life are now being reexamined. (W.F.)

When Susan asked me to come to the first meeting, I felt apprehensive. I didn't know most of the people coming. Was I getting involved in something uncomfortable, overwhelming, and possibly bigger than I wanted to deal with or commit to? Afterward I was glad I had been there, to be part of a vital group of women, an interesting, colorful, diverse group who would touch each other's lives by helping a friend. (L.T.)

CHAPTER THREE

How to Take the First Steps in Forming a Share The Care Group

You've realized that a caregiver group could be of enormous help to your sick friend. But how you approach your friend can make the difference between the idea of having a group and the reality of putting one together.

Sick People Often Resist Help

One of the biggest obstacles you may face in helping a person who is seriously ill is the person himself.

At the beginning, it is usually difficult for that person to accept all the concern flowing his way. Most of us are not used to so much caring. Many of us never had it, even when we were children, and like any new experience, it takes some getting used to. People who have had caregiver families have expressed shock that there were so many people who wanted to help, have insisted that they didn't deserve so much attention, and have been overwhelmed by the creativity, ingenuity, and depth of the caring.

They will tell you they are so exhausted from having to cope with their lives and their illness that they've lost touch with their friends. They will be sure that the people they know wouldn't want to do it. They will worry about assembling a group who don't know each other, worry that no one will come through.

When Susan was asked to assemble a group, it seemed impossible. Susan was feisty, skeptical, and stubborn. After all, she had lived through three surgeries and four courses of radiation without anyone in her company's knowing, and had even managed to be promoted.

She had fired a doctor and fought with nurses and technicians. She had kept the details of her illness from the two children who lived with her as well as most of her friends. She was critical, sharp, quick-witted, a fighter who believed she would beat this illness and regarded the surgeries and radiation treatments as "interruptions" to her life. She clung fiercely to her high-powered job and to her independence.

She argued with Dr. Miller for months, and her arguments were good ones. She was so exhausted by having to cope with her stressful job as well as her cancer that she had lost touch with a lot of her friends. She was sure the people she knew wouldn't want to do it. She worried no one would come to a meeting, let alone a meeting with a therapist. But the problems of her care soon became bigger than her arguments and she finally agreed to call her friends and acquaintances.

She was astounded when twelve of us showed up for a three-hour meeting on one day's notice.

They Believe No One Can Help

Most seriously ill people believe no one can do anything to help, and it's not surprising. They've been given horrendous diagnoses, been wheeled under huge frightening machines, and been confronted by a confusing set of options for treatments and drugs by a high-tech, overburdened medical establishment that can be impersonal and cold. They've had doctors tell them that even they may not be able to help. They feel suddenly alone, different from everyone else. When what they're facing is so huge, so catastrophic, they can't imagine it could help just to have someone to talk to, someone to go to a doctor with them, someone to hold their hand. Maybe they were never very well taken care of when they were young, so they don't believe anyone *can* take care of them.

They Fear Losing Control

Another reason they may not want help is the fear of losing control. Maybe they've survived other tragedies by retaining control. Maybe they've never confronted the fact that one day we will all lose control. In our fast-paced, chaotic, demanding world, most of us have spent years trying to gain control over our lives. We build fences and fortresses, put in alarm systems, and amass fortunes to protect ourselves. We live in a culture that tries to control the climate with air-conditioning; the sun with SPF; aging with diets, vitamins, and cosmetic surgery; the mind with meditation; the future with astrologers; the personality with drugs. To be suddenly told we have a fatal disease and must immediately have surgery and radiation or we will die, to confront the random mystery of cancer or AIDS or Alzheimer's, is at odds with everything we have been told, everything we would like to believe.

Furthermore, the idea that we can no longer take care of ourselves brings up our deepest fears and our deepest wounds. We all want to take care of ourselves. From our first step to our first bicycle to our first job, we are proud of being able to support ourselves, to contribute, to be part of things. Suddenly we feel we may no longer be useful or needed.

Asking for help means admitting how sick we are, and people with a serious illness have so many doctors' appointments, so many trips to the hospital, so many crises, that they would have to ask and ask and ask. Every time they ask they feel more helpless, more out of control. Every time they ask, they feel they are imposing on their friends and driving them away.

They Fear Losing Their Privacy

There are other fears. Most of us value our privacy and we fear that if we let a group into our lives, we will lose it. We won't have our space. They will find out our secrets. Many people are uncomfortable in groups, preferring one-on-one situations. Usually, people who are ill have come to rely heavily on one or two people and, being obsessed with their own tragedy (understandably), have no idea what a burden they have become. So the idea of a whole group coming into their life, their home, even with the best intentions, may be viewed by the sick person as loss of that one special caregiver.

They may feel that the group would bond together, leaving them out, or even be against them.

Approaching People Who Are Ill About a Caregiver Group

If You're a Friend

Assure them the group is there to help them. Tell them the group will be formed around their specific needs. The group will be made up of people who love them and want the best for them. Explain that they will have more quality time with the people closest to them because the errands, the work, and the stress will be shared by a number of people. Tell them that they will have to ask for help less often and yet more of their needs will be met.

Be honest. Above all, if you have been one of the primary caregivers and you are burning out, be honest about your own needs and feelings. Tell them you can no longer do this alone, that other people have offered to help and that *you need help* so you can go on helping them. They probably already feel guilty about asking for so much from you, and they may be relieved when you tell them the truth. It has gotten hard, you are committed, you love them, and you think you've found a way to make it easier.

If You're a Spouse or Blood Relative

If you're a husband or wife or mother or daughter, you may have a harder time asking for help or allowing others to help than your sick wife or son or mother has. One of the biggest reasons for this is what the psychologists call "denial." To let help in is to admit there's a problem. As long as no one else knows, we can tell ourselves maybe it will go away. Maybe the doctors made a mistake. Maybe we should get another opinion.

When someone we love is seriously ill, it's easy to go into denial with them. Even the medical establishment falls into this trap sometimes. One of the people we created a caregiver family for was told by her doctor not to join support groups because it would make her feel too much like a victim, that she should stay strong and she would beat her cancer. A year later, she died.

After a major shock, such as an accident or diagnosis of a serious illness, we often go into denial to protect ourselves from feeling the full impact all at once. This can be useful for a time. But don't let it keep you and the sick person from getting the help you both need.

Before you can deal with the patient's denial, you may have to deal with your own. If people are telling you you're not yourself, if people keep offering help and you keep refusing it, if you find it harder and harder to talk to doctors, if you're isolating yourself from your own friends, if you don't want to talk about it when your sick husband or sister or child does, you may be in denial, and you may need some help yourself.

But if you're clear that you need help, while your loved ones say they don't, that everything will be fine and all they need is you, you may have to tell them that you love them but you can't (or don't want to) do this alone. At this point, it may be helpful to share with them the concept of a caregiver group and even parts of this book. Above all, you must be honest about it—first with yourself, and then with them.

Approaching the Biological Family About a Caregiver Group If You're a Friend

If you're a close friend of the person who is ill, you may spend more time with him than anyone else does. You may live next door, while his mother and father live in another state. You may know his other friends and see how a group could come together. But you must consider the feelings of the biological family.

People in your friend's real family may be too proud to ask for help. Many of us equate asking for help with weakness. A husband may want to feel he can take care of his own wife, or vice versa. A devoted mother may not want a group taking care of her son or daughter. A family may not want strangers watching them or meddling in their affairs.

So it's important to include them from the very beginning and to assure them that the group will in no way interfere in their lives or take their place. Instead, the group will remove some of the stress they're under so that they can spend more quality family time together.

No matter how difficult it seemed at the beginning, the biological families were always happy that the Share The Care family was there. Here are some quotes from Susan's real family.

From her daughters:

People really want to help. The [group] is the best way. It helps the immediate family feel supported and less overwhelmed. It shows the person who is ill that you really care about them and makes them feel supported as well, especially at a time when the person and/or family feels so helpless.

As a young person, I would encourage you to try to be in touch with [caregiver group] members that you know and are close to so you feel like part of the group and the whole process. Remember the group is there to help you as well as your parent. It will help you be part of what is happening to your parent and be more in control of your own life. It can only improve your relationship with your parent as well as reduce your own confusion and fear.

From her parents:

At first I felt guilty living in Florida and not being able to be with Susan. But I met some of the group soon after it was formed. I couldn't help falling in love with them. I knew she was in good hands and felt no resentment.

Knowing Susan had her [caregiver] family all the time gave us relief from anxiety and allowed us to carry on our own lives. In fact, we adopted all you girls as part of our family.

Approaching People to Be in Your Caregiver Group

The most important thing to stress when you approach people about being in your group is the fact that they will be *part of a group*, that no one person will have to do it all and that no one will have to do things they're not good at, afraid of, or simply don't want to do.

Tell them about the other people who have already agreed to be in the group. They may have met or know some of them already. Tell them there is a system that will make it easy for them to help and easier for the person who is ill to accept their help. Acknowledge their goodness for wanting to help and tell them how excited you are personally about their being in the group.

The Special Benefits of Being Part of a Caregiver Group

When we held our first meeting with Dr. Miller, one of the questions she asked was "What do each of you think you can get personally, just for yourself, by being in this group?" At the time, most of us thought she was crazy. Some of us were even offended. We were there to help Susan, not ourselves.

But Dr. Miller insisted. In fact, she even had us do an exercise called "What's in It for You?" It was hard for us to think of things to write. Most of us said things like "It will be nice to be a part of something that does good for someone" and "This will be a way for me to give back some of the good things I've received." Then Susan's daughter Keri changed the course of the exercise when she said she was grateful to have the group "so I won't feel so guilty about not being able to take care of my mom." It was a brave thing for her to say because it was so honest. Then other people thought a little harder. Someone said, "I've always wanted a child and wasn't able to have one, so this will give me a chance to nurture and mother someone." Someone else surprised us all by saying "Now I'll get to spend more time with Susan."

Three years later, when Susan's group met with Francine and her friends, we asked them to share what they thought they might get out of being in Francine's group. They were as perplexed by the question as we had once been, and they shared similar thoughts. But when we shared what we actually got out of being in Susan's caregiver family, they were amazed at the depth of our responses.

I discovered I had an inner strength and love I didn't know was there. I was able to break through my own fears and be there for my friend. I learned to put aside personal differences with other members of the family and to confront any issue. As a captain [the role of a "captain" will be explained in chapter 8], I had to delegate responsibilities to other members and make sure they followed through. Most of all, I learned that love and caring rise above all else. (A.R.)

I am better able to relate to people who are ill. I'm not as fearful of keeping in contact or just calling to see how they are. (T.C.)

I have developed a new philosophy about my own life. I'm freer, more vocal, more daring, interested in many more things. I am enjoying life more. (J.W.)

I've never been in a group before. This was a very focused group that had a mission, but that mission embraced us all as we took care of each other as well as Susan. (C.V.)

As people played their unique roles in caring for someone else, their priorities seemed to shift from reasoning to trusting, from revering the intellect to revering the mystery, from looking good to doing good, from living in the future or the past to living in the moment, and from accomplishment to meaning.

Some people said they felt more connected to humanity. Some said they began to see how we all share the same fears, needs, and desires. Others felt they got a sense of their own place in the world—a sense of belonging. They found out more about their own strengths and weaknesses and they began to acknowledge the strengths and accept the weaknesses. They realized that having limits doesn't mean you're bad or weak, or that the job won't get done.

One person said, "I stopped taking myself quite so seriously and stopped complaining about the small stuff. At the same time, I took myself more seriously. I began to know I could be counted on, and what I was doing really meant something."

So when you're thinking about asking people to be in a caregiver group, don't think it's all sacrifice, pain, and sadness. Remember to tell them it's also about friendship, meaning, and miracles.

> I never felt I had anything to offer people, but now I know I do have something to give. (T.M.)

> Facing something as terrifying as cancer is a very scary thing, especially since my father and stepmother died of cancer. But . . . it feels good to help someone you like. . . . It also puts my own problems in perspective for me. (F.S.)

> I thought by being part of "another's struggle," it would take me away from my inner struggles. I would open up my life to fear, emotion, responsibility. I would let something else in my life and not run away and immerse myself in my work. I was right, and my life blossomed in a way I never dreamed. (L.L.)

CHAPTER FOUR

How to Use This Book

In the next section of this book (part 2) you will find a step-by-step guide to forming your own caregiver group. We suggest you read through it once, finish the rest of the book, and then come back and spend some time with part 2. It consists of six areas.

Many people use the book as a reference handbook over time, dipping back into specific chapters as needed.

1. Assessing the Sick Person's Needs

Before you hold your first group meeting, you need to know exactly what the sick person needs, and in some cases what their spouses, children, or parents need.

In part 2 you'll find a set of questions to help you identify the kinds of skills you need and to give you a realistic idea of the kind of commitment required by your group.

2. Holding Your Share The Care Meeting

This meeting is the foundation of every caregiver group. In part 2 you will learn what you need, how to begin, whom to invite, and how to explain the concept so people understand it and want to come to the meeting. Part 2 also explains in great detail what you have to do to lead a meeting.

We have tried to help you create the meeting in such a way that you feel we are in the room with you and that it is absolutely safe for the person who is ill and everyone there to share their feelings. The initial meeting may seem like a big challenge, but it will come together even if you've never conducted a meeting in your life.

3. Doing a Tried-and-True Set of Exercises

There are eleven exercises that seem to get every caregiver group off to the right start. They have worked for many groups, so we have tried to give them to you in great detail. We have laid out the amount of time each takes, the purpose of each, and the materials you will need.

4. Putting Practical Systems in Place

There are also several practical systems we discovered during our three and a half years of caring for Susan, and we share them with you to use in the second half of the meeting. There is a system for collecting and coordinating information and keeping your group informed and up-to-date. There is a system for making sure someone is always in charge but no one is overburdened. There is also a system for making sure you have the right person for each job, and one to ensure that the person who is ill never has to deal with logistics or group issues but can concentrate totally on getting well.

One person cited some of the problems a group had before it put the systems into play:

- There were about three people who were on call twenty-four hours a day and they were falling apart.
- Everyone would show up at the hospital or no one would show up. The doctors would get upset because at times we'd have eight people in the room.
- People didn't know how to help.
- Some people weren't good at certain jobs and would end up staying away altogether.
- Guilt drove everyone. No one knew how to help in a productive way. (D.R.)

5. Using the Workbook

At the end of the meeting section is the workbook. The workbook contains updated forms and instructions we originally created to keep Susan's Funny Family organized and running smoothly. In an effort to save you time and energy, we have made all of the forms in the book available to be downloaded, edited, and printed out for immediate use from the book Web site: http://www.sharethecare.org. The book also contains blank forms that can be photocopied if you have no Internet access.

The difference this type of organization can make on the process of caregiving was explained by a member this way:

> Having lived through lung cancer with my husband I know firsthand how exhausting (mentally and emotionally) caring for a seriously ill person can be. Either six people show up at the same time or no one shows up for two weeks. An organized support group brings tremendous relief to everyone. It brings stability and support on every level. (C.S.)

6. Learning the Seven Principles

During the years that Susan's Funny Family was in operation, certain issues came up again and again. In dealing with these issues, we discovered there were some guiding principles that seemed to hold our group together through the good times and the bad. They were somehow the keys to our ability to work together and they proved themselves over and over. We call them the Seven Principles, and as you prepare to take part in a caregiver group, we urge you to keep these points in mind:

Principle 1: Sharing Responsibility Is the Key to Not Burning Out.

- No one person has to be in charge all the time.
- No one person has to deal with every crisis.
- No one person has to be on call every single day.
- No one person has to make all the decisions, all the time.

- No one person has to try to run his own life plus the entire, complex life of his loved one.
- Let the others do their share. They want to. They need to.

Principle 2: It Won't Work Unless Everyone Gains Something Personally.

- Recognize the importance of personal rewards.
- The patient will feel too guilty unless you gain something too.

Principle 3: Know Your Limits and Stick to Them.

- Whatever you can do to help is enough.
- If you can't or don't want to do something, don't. (Someone else is probably good at it, or loves to do it.)

Principle 4: There's No One Right Way to Do It.

- If there are ten members, there will be ten ways to do it.
- It's okay to disagree.
- Agree on basics, then follow the rules. You may learn some amazing things.

Principle 5: Anyone Who Wants to Help Should Be Encouraged.

- A group needs eight, but ten is better.
- If the main caregivers are "real" family, they must be willing to broaden the circle.
- "Free-floaters" (people who can help only occasionally) are very important.

Principle 6: Trust the Group; Support Each Other.

- The group has power.
- Someone has the talent or the answer.
- Go on vacation. The others are there.

- Share your feelings; share the goal.
- Spend time together; acknowledge each other.

Principle 7: Keep Your Own Life in Good Working Order.

- Take care of yourself, or you won't be able to take care of the patient.
- Exercise, rest, stay "in life."
- Lighten the rest of your load.
- Don't forget about your own family and friends.
- Let your friends, your boss, and your own family know what you are doing.

PART 2

Starting Your Group and Making It Run

CHAPTER FIVE

A Message from the Authors: How to Use This Section

The next four chapters are the nitty-gritty of group caregiving. We have tried to spell it out from beginning to end as best we could. In chapter 1, we explained the concept of Share The Care. In chapter 2, we tried to help you determine if this approach would work for you and talked about the benefits of "sharing the care." In chapter 3, we explained how to approach the person who is ill and the people who might be in your group. Now you will see the specific steps to take to create your group and get it working. We've talked about the personal rewards of being in a caregiver group. Now you will find an exercise that helps the members of the group get in touch with what exactly they might get just for themselves. We've talked about the seven principles behind every caregiver group's success. Now you will see how to create an environment that will begin to focus everyone on the same goal and bond them together as a group.

Assessing the Sick Person's Needs

Before you hold your first group meeting, you need to know exactly what the sick person needs—and in some cases what the spouse, children, or parents need. By answering the following questions, you will begin to identify the kinds of skills your group could use and you will get a realistic idea of the kind of commitment required by your group.

1. How Quickly Do You Need to Get Organized?

If your friend has had a sudden stroke or an accident, you will obviously have to get your group mobilized as quickly and as efficiently as possible. But while a temporary need may require immediate action, it may not require a long-term commitment.

2. What Is the Time Frame of Commitment?

If the person who is sick has a complex, serious illness, it may require a long-term commitment from the group members. It will also require a great deal of strength to cope with the emotional ups and downs. In this case, you may want to assemble a fairly large group. It is easier to handle a long-term commitment if you are sharing the responsibilities and can keep your own life in good order. This was the case with Susan's group. Her cancer progressed slowly over several years, causing a gradual deterioration of her physical capabilities and eventually her death. We had twelve full-time members and many free-floaters, and we never felt we had too many people. Many groups today average around twenty to twenty-five members, while some have even had as many as sixty people.

On the other hand, perhaps your sick friend has a short-term illness and has been assured of recovery within a certain time frame. Such people may need a great deal of help, but only for a short time. Their emotional needs will not be as great because they know they're going to get better. If that's the case, a small group may be able to handle the situation without burning out.

If the person who is sick has a terminal illness, you may not know how long you will need the group, but you do know you will need people who can be committed to someone very ill, someone they are probably going to lose, people who are willing to make those final days, weeks, months, or even years as rewarding and comfortable as possible.

3. What Are the Physical and Mental States of the Sick Person?

Are they physically handicapped? Are they temporarily or permanently disabled? Are they becoming slowly disabled and having difficulty coping with everyday activities? Are they using a cane or a walker or do they need to be in a wheelchair? They may require help only with such physically demanding chores as cleaning and shopping, or they may require help with such personal tasks as taking baths or washing their hair. Do they need more help than they are willing to admit?

Perhaps they are physically strong but unable to communicate and understand what is happening. Perhaps they cannot be left alone. If this is the case (as with Alzheimer's disease), a large group will be beneficial even if it includes many free-floaters who can commit to only small amounts of time.

Perhaps they are still in shock or in denial about what has happened to them and they need a moral support system and a sense they are not alone. Do they need emotional support when going to doctors' appointments and treatments? Do they need perseverance and a cheering section to keep going? Do they need a sense of peace and understanding and permission to finally stop fighting their illness and let go?

4. Does the Sick Person Have a Spouse or Family?

Does a husband, wife, roommate, or child need support? Are they burnt out from trying to deal with their loved one's illness alone? If there is no spouse, will someone from the biological family be living with the patient? Is the family willing to become part of the caregiver group?

Does the patient have children? Do the group members know the patient's children really well? If not, it would be helpful if some of the people in the caregiver group were parents, so they could understand and support the children of the sick person. If the sick person doesn't have to worry about his or her children, he or she can better focus on healing.

Does the sick person have a dog or cat or parrot or goldfish? A pet is often overlooked when illness strikes. Yet a pet may be an important part of the healing process. Who within your caregiver group can take charge of or share in the care of the family pet?

5. What Are the Logistical Problems of the Sick Person?

Does the patient live in a rural area where your group would have to travel long distances just to get to him? Will you need cars or an ambulette service? Will people need to arrange to stay overnight?

Does the sick person live in a big city but his friends live out of town, or vice versa? Does the group need to learn a subway system or bus routes? Do they need a map to get to the person's home?

Will the sick person be making long trips to distant hospitals for treatments or to a specialist in another city or even to an alternative care program in another state or country? How can the group deal with these requirements?*

A Caregiver Group Officially Begins with Its First Meeting

Now that you have an idea of what you might need, you are ready to hold your first meeting. In the next four chapters, we have spelled out everything we did and said at our first meeting and in subsequent meetings. We have tried to cover all the issues that might come up. We have given tips to the people leading the meeting. The workbook section is designed so you can download the forms from the book Web site and print or photocopy them so everyone can have a copy. This will enable you to get the group going quickly and easily.

The first meeting is a courageous beginning, a scary time, a time for asking for help, and a loving time. Each first meeting is different in tone. Some are hyperefficient, some very emotional, some quiet, and some stormy, but most are a combination of all these things. Regardless of the tone, the efficiency, or the emotionality of your first meeting, the first key element of all meetings is a series of tried-and-true group exercises. The second key element of all meetings is the workbook. The third key element, and the most important, is the strong commitment of two people, whom we call the leader and the coordinator.

* See "Caregiving Far from Home" on page 200 for important information on this issue.

They are the two people who will set up and lead everyone else through the meeting. The most important qualification for them both is commitment to creating a caregiver group. Once the group has been formed, there will be many people to share in the tasks of caregiving, but before the first meeting it will be the leader and the coordinator who will create the initial energy and enthusiasm, who will help the sick person and his or her loved ones see the need for a group, and who will find the people who care and convince them to come to the first meeting.

If you find you are the only one with that kind of commitment, whether or not you feel you could be the leader or coordinator, *we strongly suggest that before you try to do this alone you find a partner who will help you,* even at this early stage. Do not try to assume both roles yourself.

The jobs of the leader and the coordinator are quite different from each other, as you will see in the next three chapters, but both jobs are equally important.

Choosing the Leader

The leader should be someone who is comfortable talking to people and sharing feelings, and someone who is good at listening. The leader must be able to talk openly and honestly with the person who is ill and must be comfortable with the idea of approaching people to be in the group.

The leader is responsible for leading people through the exercises in the first part of the meeting and the later exercises that begin to bond people together, and for keeping the meeting emotionally on track.

If you cannot allow uncomfortable feelings to be expressed because you are too upset, too close to the person who is sick, too distracted, or too burnt out, don't take on the job of leader. Let someone else do it. He or she may not have the same emotional responses as you.

Choosing the Coordinator

The coordinator should be someone who is very reliable, who is good at paperwork, is organized, and is a clear communicator. The coordinator should have a computer and printer since he or she will be counted on to collect information during the meeting, organize it, copy it, and mail it to all members within a week. If the group has fifteen members or more, try to recruit an assistant coordinator to help with organizing and distributing information following the meeting.

If you are already overworked and have little time in your schedule, don't take on this job.

While the leader may be the one to break the ice and get the meeting going, it is often the coordinator who keeps it going and untangles it when it gets bogged down. While the leader creates the possibility and sets the emotional tone for the meeting, it is the coordinator who makes it a practical reality, and it is the leader and coordinator working together who make true group caregiving possible.

Mastering the Exercises

Unfortunately, if you are going to be either the leader or the coordinator, you cannot just pick up this book at the meeting and read from it.

You must spend time studying the exercises and practicing them. Although it may sound silly, we strongly recommend that you read the exercises aloud and that you pretend you have a group in front of you when you do it.

Try to imagine all the people you've invited to the meeting sitting in a circle around you. In your mind's eye, see the person who is ill in the group as well. Rehearse your part as you go along. Both the leader and the coordinator must know the exercises well. To do this takes spending time together.

Mastering the Forms

Both the leader and the coordinator must have a good working knowledge of how to fill in the forms (discussed and explained in the next few chapters). A trick we have found that greatly accelerates learning the forms (which at first may seem overwhelming but really are quite simple) is to practice with them. Unlike the exercises, where you must use your imagination to best prepare, the forms are easily mastered when both the leader and the coordinator take the time to fill them out *as if they were in the situation the form addresses.*

Both rehearsing the exercises and filling in the forms will take some time, but we have found that for every five minutes you spend in this preparation, you can avoid twenty minutes of chaos and confusion at the time of your first meeting. You do not have to do your first meeting perfectly, but you must do it carefully.

Finding the Words to Say

Sometimes, no matter how well you have rehearsed your part, the emotions of a first meeting may leave you tongue-tied. It is for this reason that we have given you a suggested script to follow as you go along. It is just a suggestion and a friendly backup. We encourage you to use your own words and your own style. Don't be afraid to use your sense of humor or to show your compassion or wisdom. The more comfortable you are with the exercises and forms, the easier and more personal your meeting will be. *Feel free to modify our chart systems to work for you and your group.*

We wish you the best of luck. It is our hope that when your first meeting ends, you will have all the emotional grounding and practical tools you need and that your Share The Care family will be empowered as a caregiver group that will be able to handle almost anything.

CHAPTER SIX

Planning the Meeting: Getting Started

How to Begin

You begin with a list, a phone, two possible meeting dates, and a place to hold the meeting. If you're the leader or the coordinator, your first job is to sit with the person who is ill and compile a list of the names and phone numbers of their friends, acquaintances, and biological family members.

Whom to Invite to the Meeting

When you meet with the person who is ill, encourage that person not to censor anyone who may want to help. Ask them to think of work friends, school friends, friends who shared hobbies or community activities, friends from their church or synagogue. Find out what groups they belong to, who their neighbors are. Ask about the people they work with, or used to work with. Encourage them to talk about the people who have been important in their lives.

They may be reluctant at first, and you may want to go through their address book with them. You might suggest going through their e-mail addresses, their Palm Pilot, their office Rolodex, their college yearbook, even their Christmas card list. Ask about relatives. If they have a biological family, be sure to invite them to the first meeting.

Don't make judgments about who can and cannot be in the group. Give a sixteen-year-old daughter a real responsibility. Don't assume that a ten-year-old can't do anything. Take a neighbor up on her offer to cook.

What about the college roommate who just moved back to the city? The girlfriend who always wanted to be a nurse but went into business instead? The person in the office who is always trying to be a friend? The old friend who just moved back into town and doesn't know anybody?

Don't Ignore Part-Timers, Latecomers, or People Who Live Far Away

A caregiver group works best with ten to twelve full members, but the people we called "free-floaters" (people who couldn't be full-time members) were often the ones who stepped in and saved the day with an extra phone call, an extra visit, an extra dinner, an available car.

Susan's caregiver group also had people who joined long after we first went into operation.

> I never knew Susan as a physically healthy person. She was in the middle of the cancer battle when we met at Omega, the new-age summer camp for grown-ups, where she was taking a writing course, determined to write the story of her Funny Family. To me, Susan was a brave warrior enlisting her nearest and dearest as part of her troop. I was therefore honored to become a part of this as the newest member. In the course of belonging to the Funny Family, I felt blessed to be part of something that was at its very source about humanity, simplicity, grace. (S.N.)

Don't neglect people who live in other towns, even if they're some distance away. We had one honorary member who lived thousands of miles away. He was one of Susan's oldest and dearest friends and was as much a part of Susan's Funny Family schedule as the people who lived right next door. His constant and regular phone calls gave Susan a great deal of strength, and his help in writing her story as a screenplay helped to make her feel a part of life until the very end.

> I was three thousand miles from Susan and the Funny Family. My only contact with her was our frequent and sometimes lengthy phone conver-

sations. I felt since this was my only chance to help, I couldn't back away from the issue. Pull my punches, so to speak. Consequently, our conversations were very meaningful, even from a distance. (B.T.)

During the time your group is in operation, you will discover that "help" has many faces and many forms, that people who seemed frightened may turn out to have untold strengths, that a daughter can be very grown-up, a neighbor very comforting, and most of all that if you are about to cope with a long-term, complex illness, you need all the help you can get. Susan's group had twelve. Francine's group had twenty-four. There have been groups with as few as eight and as many as one hundred. No group ever said they had too many people to help.

Finding the People Who Care

On the following pages is a list that may help people who are ill find the people for their unique caregiver group. If you go through the list with them, you will find that there are many people who care. People you never heard of. People you never expected. People who feel just like you do—they want to help, but they don't know how. Even if there are items on the list that do not apply to your friend, the list is sure to spark additional ideas.

Encourage both men and women, children and the elderly, close friends and casual acquaintances, people who've been caregivers and people who haven't, people who want to do a lot, people who can do only a little. The more different backgrounds and abilities you have in the group, the more you'll be able to help. There are enough jobs in every caregiver group so that every man, woman, and child can find a suitable job.

Some Ideas on Where to Look

- Immediate family and all relatives (including children and teens)
- Close and not-so-close friends
- Neighbors (current and old—from another neighborhood)
- Colleagues, past and present
- Business associates
- Clients
- Unions
- Business organizations

- Church, synagogue, or meditation groups
- Fellow PTA committee members
- Classes they take (dance, art, photography, computer, sailing)
- School or university (night classes, summer classes)
- Friends from the armed services
- Old schoolmates
- Old roommates
- Fraternities, sororities
- Elks Club, Friars Club, Toastmasters, et al.
- Organizations for retired professionals in their field
- Former students
- Country club friends
- Tennis or golf partners
- Friends from yoga class or the health club
- Fellow joggers
- Friends of friends who want to help
- Priest, minister, rabbi
- Local community center
- Senior citizens center
- Rugby, soccer, basketball teammates
- Skiing friends
- Summerhouse friends
- People they know from walking the dog
- New friends
- Parents of their children's friends
- Local community theater
- State fair friends
- 4-H club
- Friends from places they have done volunteer work
- Fishing and hunting friends
- Clubs: cooking club, book club, bowling club, chess club, and so on
- Singing groups, chorus (even if they see each other only at Christmas)
- Friends' spouses, boyfriends, girlfriends
- People training for social work
- Student doctors and nurses
- Housekeeper, maid, cleaning lady, babysitter
- Hiking and camping friends
- Friends met on vacation
- Boy Scouts, Girls Scouts, service groups
- Political organizations
- Volunteer groups
- Friendly manager of the local grocery store
- Someone with nothing to do (bored with retirement)
- A pharmacist at the local drugstore
- Support-group friends
- Cancer Care, Gay Men's Health Crisis (any applicable support groups for specific problems)
- 12-step programs
- "Quit smoking" program friends
- Friends from special courses (for instance, Course in Miracles, Life-Spring)
- Friends from group therapy

Have Two Dates

The leader, coordinator, and person who is ill should agree on two dates when they are all available. Those should be the meeting dates you propose when making your calls to prospective group members.

Where to Hold the Meeting

Once you have two possible meeting dates, you will need a place to hold the meeting. Someone can volunteer his or her home or apartment. If the person who is ill is very tired or sick, you may want to have it at his or her home. It is important that the person who is ill be there if at all possible.

Wherever the meeting is held, be sure that the location is dedicated to your meeting for the whole afternoon or evening, with no interruptions, no television, no phones that have to be answered. If there are small children in the house, hire a babysitter to entertain them and keep them occupied in a different part of the house—or, better yet, at a neighbor's place.

Getting Off to the Right Start

Getting off to the right start depends on your first communication with potential members. You should contact the people on your list individually by phone rather than by e-mail. Though it is tempting to contact people the *easy way*, it is best to do this job the *personal way* so you can address any questions or fears right away. This is critical because you will be setting the tone for the whole process of coming together to help.

If you are making the calls, remember that the meeting begins the minute you say hello. Your voice should be friendly and reassuring. Be sure to take time with each person. The people you are calling have probably not been invited to a meeting like this before, and if they know how ill their friend is they may already be frightened. Start out by saying that the person who is ill suggested you call, and that you are also a friend. Ask if this is a good time for them to talk. If not, arrange a time to call back.

How to Explain

Explaining the concept is easier than you might think. Tell the person you are calling a little about what is going on with the person who is ill. Then say that you are having a meeting to form a group, and explain briefly what it is about. Say that you have found a group caregiver system called Share The Care that not only takes care of the person who is ill but also is a way for people to do exactly as much as they can to help. Tell them many groups around the country have used it with great success.

People who are close to the sick person (and have probably been doing too much) will be relieved to hear about the group. People who are casual acquaintances (and are wondering what they could do) will be glad for the opportunity. Most people will find the prospect of this meeting exciting, if a little scary, and will want to know more about it. You may want to tell them that it is not only a way to take care of your mutual friend but also a way to take care of the caregivers.* You can also refer them to the Web site at http://www.sharethecare.org, where they can read about the Share The Care system in more depth before the meeting.

Getting a Commitment

After you have introduced yourself and explained the purpose of your call, give them the two alternate dates and the address where the meeting will be held. Ask them to call you back to tell you which is the best date for them. Set a deadline within the next few days or you might wind up waiting weeks for a callback. Then you will call back confirming the date that is best for the majority of the group.

Your meeting date should be the one most people can attend. Do not have two meetings. It is important that one group be formed. Do not be concerned if forty people plan to come to this first meeting when you need only twenty. Some may not come. Others may drop out later.

Although it is time-consuming, making these phone calls is the only thing you will have to do alone, and it is the only way to ensure that you will

* Review chapter 3, "How to Take the First Steps in Forming a Share The Care Group," for advice on approaching people.

have enough people for your first, and most important, meeting. When they call back, keep a list of who's coming. You will need it later to make up name tags.

Before you hang up, thank them for their willingness to come to the meeting, express the gratitude of the person who is ill, and reiterate that you are excited about forming this group.

When You Call the Biological Family

The best time to call the biological family is after you have a leader and a coordinator and at least five people committed to coming to the meeting. When you call, explain exactly as you have done before, only this time you must add something. It is important that you tell the real family that this group is in no way replacing them. You might want to say: "When one member of a family is sick, the whole family is hurting. What we hope the group will do is to take away some of the stress so that you can all concentrate on just being a family." Assure them that the group will in no way interfere with or limit their time with their loved one, but will instead make it easier for them to just be together and not have to worry about logistics. Let them know groups around the country have been a great source of strength for "real" family members.

The Leader and Coordinator Prepare

Now that you have your meeting date and confirmations from everyone who will attend, you need to prepare your individual parts of the meeting. But first there is a job you should do together.

Identifying Your Group's Skills

Your group's power will ultimately lie in discovering, sharing, and utilizing *all* your combined abilities, experience, and knowledge. One of your jobs in your first meeting is to try to identify what these abilities are.

For example, a member who works in a supermarket might easily handle large shopping orders. An accountant could be the person to call for balancing the checkbook or dealing with taxes. A saleswoman in a department store would be able to do some personal shopping and make returns if needed. The weekend carpenter might be the person to fix something in need of repair in the home.

To help you assess your group, we have tried to pinpoint below several types of member skills we found invaluable in Susan's group.

Assistant Coordinator

If you have more than fifteen people, the coordinator will need someone to help organize all the information you collect. Sandy, a member of Susan's group who lived some distance away and was not able to participate on a weekly basis, turned out to be a crack assistant. We will never forget the day Sandy mailed a computer printout of our Yellow Pages information. It made a huge difference because none of us had a computer at that time, and it got the group off to a grand official start.

Today, most of us have computers, and it is just a question of who is good at this. The assistant coordinator could be responsible for all charts that need to be downloaded and edited (Yellow Pages, or the Rotating Captains Schedule). If some new type of chart is required, perhaps the assistant has a program in his or her computer that can make the job a cinch. The assistant should be a detail-oriented, well-organized person.

The assistant coordinator can be a free-floater (a part-time member) who is called upon from time to time with a specific job request. He or she can live in another town or state, as Sandy did, since the information can be sent electronically or by snail mail.

The Researcher

Today the medical field is so specialized and serious illnesses are so complex that sick person and the family need specialized research in order to make important decisions about treatments, alternative care, or other issues. Let's say your friend wanted to know all about the various treatment centers around the country that dealt with his specific illness. This could be a long and tedious job unless the person doing it really enjoyed this kind of challenge. Such a person would be willing to spend time researching sites on the Internet. This job may also require following leads; talking to strangers on the phone; asking questions and getting referrals; and accumulating and downloading information on locations, costs, living facilities, references, and requirements. The researcher should be someone who is not satisfied until he or she has all the facts needed.

The researcher would pull together, sort through, and print out all the relevant information for the patient to review. After the patient reviews it, the researcher might go back for more details, if necessary, once the list has been narrowed down to two or three possibilities.

If time is of the essence and research is needed quickly, divide this job among several people so it is manageable, and then have them put it together for review. If the patient is too ill to read it, a small core group of family, or closest confidants should review it for discussion with the patient. If at all possible, get input from a nurse, doctor, or other practitioner with medical training.

The Arranger

There are probably several people in your group who are natural arrangers. Perhaps they have their own businesses or oversee a large number of employees. They're good at organizing huge projects by quickly assessing all the possibilities and options, and they're great at details, delegating responsibility, and following through.

Barbara K. was such an arranger in our group. Working with Susan, she made all the arrangements for the wedding of Susan's younger daughter, Elissa, during the last year of Susan's life.

This job included getting invitations and announcements done, finding a location, arranging for the ceremony, overseeing costs, setting the menu, and ordering the cake and the flowers. Barbara, who was also involved in her husband's business, was similar to Susan in her practical, no-nonsense approach to things. Susan instinctively felt comfortable that Barbara would get the best place for the best price at the best time available, and she did.

What major job needs to be done for your friend? Maybe they have a son or daughter about to interview for colleges in several widespread locations. Or perhaps their children are going to summer camp and need someone to organize them and drive them two hundred miles and get them settled.

Just look around . . . Has someone done this before with her own kids? Maybe two people could share the job.

The Experienced Caregiver

In our group, there were several members who had taken care of a parent or relative (though none had ever taken care of a peer or friend), and much of this experience came into play and helped all of us when Susan got progressively worse.

At one point, several of us discussed Susan's decline as she took to her bed. We sensed a subtle change in her, and we knew things were moving into an area where we would need more assistance from a professional source. One of our members had dealt with a hospice when her father (who suffered with cancer) was moved to one during the last weeks of his illness. She could not express the extent of her thankfulness for having had their help at a very difficult time.

Because of her experience, two of us went to visit a hospice to collect information and to understand exactly what it is a hospice does, how it works, and when we would need one. This visit helped to relieve some of our own fears, and later we were able to discuss hospice help with Susan intelligently when the need for it was confirmed by her doctor.

Ask questions, talk to members about their past caregiving efforts, and acknowledge and learn from them.

The Chief Cook and Bottlewasher

This could be a neighbor, a co-worker, the friend down the block. She's usually a part-time member who's not listed on the weekly schedule that will be drawn up. It's the person who says "I'm going to the store. Do you need anything?" Or "I was baking bread anyway, so I baked some for you."

Often, these unique members don't consider themselves important because they're not involved in going to hospitals or doctors or making big decisions. They don't give themselves credit for what they contribute on a daily basis.

Within our group, Susan had a neighbor, Eileen M., who collected mail, ran errands, cooked little treats for her on a daily basis, and often served gourmet meals to whoever was visiting. She always insisted that it was nothing, saying she was cooking for herself anyway, but to Susan she was a godsend.

Remember, if you have neighbor members (who help out on a daily basis), remind them how important what they do is to the group. (Your friend may be so absorbed in his illness he may not thank them anymore.) Acknowledge your entire cast; every player loves a little applause now and then.

The Creative Types

There were a few artist types in Susan's group. They brought flowers, photographs, crystals, paintings, and numerous other things to make Susan's surroundings more soothing and pleasant. Jill was one of the more entertaining members of our group; she always had a funny story and could make Susan laugh under the worst of circumstances. Others came armed with music to play or DVDs to watch.

If, for example, your friend has temporarily (or permanently) lost his or her eyesight and can no longer stand the drone of the television set or the music selection on the radio, is there a group member who is an actor, a writer, or who is blessed with a great voice? Assign this person the job of reading aloud as a form of entertainment or education for the person who is ill.

Encourage your members to think of ways to make life a little more pleasant for someone who literally can't get out there and smell the roses.

The Member with a Special Skill

A group will most likely have a member with some special skill that could be a real blessing at some time during the patient's illness.

Pat was the sister of one of our regular members. She was also a registered nurse. Pat didn't know Susan that well, but she pitched in several times and lent her expertise after several of Susan's surgeries. She served as a private duty nurse and was able to be in the recovery room with Susan right after surgery. It was so reassuring to Susan, who was terrified of operations, to see a friendly face she knew when she first opened her eyes.

Maybe your group has an attorney who could execute a will or oversee a power of attorney. Is there an insurance expert who could get you through complicated paperwork and red tape? A nutritionist who could plan a balanced diet and recommend vitamin supplements or health drinks? Maybe you have a hairdresser in your group who could help your friend find the perfect wig *before* she starts chemotherapy.

The Shopper

The shopper is someone who loves the challenge of finding whatever it is you need (clothes, equipment, household items). Such people know every nook and cranny of the shopping mall, and to them shopping is not a job—it's a kind of treasure hunt.

Barbara D. was such a person in Susan's group. She had good taste, was well organized, and knew exactly what she was looking for and where to find it. She had a talent for finding great bargains and would cheerfully make returns if something wasn't quite right.

Perhaps your sick friend's three children need new school clothes but the person is too sick to take them shopping. The shopper could consult with your friend, determine a budget, decide what is needed, get the correct sizes. She could even take the children shopping with her.

Perhaps someone in your group is a salesperson in a department store and can work with the shopper and even get discounts. Don't overlook the shopper; he or she is a very valuable group member.

The Handyman, Handywoman, or Weekend Carpenter

You know the type. No matter what they do for a living, they love to putter in their workshop or garage and can repair anything. They own every tool in existence. They can fix a leak (at least until the plumber gets there). They can start a car in any weather, set up the new DVD and sound system, put up the screens, and take down the storm windows. They have a ladder and a drill. They can clean out the drains and roof gutters, and they know exactly whom to call if they can't do something. If you have one of these types in your group (man or woman, full-time member or free-floater), he or she can be indispensable, especially when you are making safety or comfort adjustments to your friend's home.*

The Tutor

Perhaps the person who is ill is a single parent, and now there is no one to help with the children's homework, no one to keep them interested and excited about learning while their parent recovers. Or perhaps the person who is ill is a child and has to stay home from school while getting better. Who can give children the special attention they need during these difficult times?

Is there a teacher, substitute teacher, student teacher, or retired teacher among the rank and file of your group? If so, such a person could be of great help to a sick child or to the children of a sick parent.

The Driver

Don't underestimate the person in your group who has a car, loves to drive, and is good at directions. Myrna was the official driver of Susan's group and was a great comfort to Susan. People traveling to hospitals or to their first chemotherapy appointment and people in rural areas who have to travel long distances just to get to the doctor are under enough stress without worrying about road maps, bad weather, and getting lost. A competent, willing driver can greatly reduce their stress and make the trip easier.

The Child

Children can be a great blessing as part of a caregiver group. They can bring life and laughter into a sick person's home and can give the person who is seriously ill a much-needed lift with their cheery smiles and bright eyes.

There are many jobs children can do. They can walk the dog, pick up the mail, feed the cat, deliver food, rake the leaves, mow the lawn, return a

* See chapter 17, "Making the Home Safe and Comfortable," for specific information.

video, buy a newspaper, water the plants, pick the vegetables, take out the garbage. They will benefit greatly from having a real responsibility and from understanding the importance of their jobs. Take their help seriously and acknowledge them as part of the caregiver group.

The Teen

Today's teens are involved in all kinds of volunteering. From participating in Walks for Cures to selling cakes for charity, they are taking an active role in making their school, community, and world a better place. Instinctively, they know there is no finer way to learn compassion, understanding, and kindness than by helping another person.

Teens can do all kinds of jobs from errands to house chores. For a family with young children, a teen can handle babysitting or coaching young kids on their soccer moves. A teen can also provide comfort to an elderly person by helping them around the house or yard or teaching them how to explore the Internet. They can bring a smile to the face of a fellow teen with cancer as they recount how their high school won the state football championship. Watch their confidence bloom as they discover the true meaning of "making a difference."

The Elder Citizen

An older person may be waiting for an opportunity to help but may feel as if there's nothing he or she can do. Or people may be afraid to ask them, fearing they're not up to it, when all along they want very much to feel needed. Older people have a great deal of wisdom about life and death and can be of enormous psychological support to a seriously ill person. They may only be able to do lighter jobs and they may take a little longer. On the other hand, they may surprise everyone with the skills they have accumulated over a lifetime.

Suggest that your sick friend's eighty-year-old aunt bake some of her famous oatmeal cookies. Offer to go out and get the ingredients. Ask the senior citizen who lives next door if he would water the lawn once a week, or just look in on the person who is ill. Susan's Uncle Sid was known to fill in when we needed extra help.

. . .

Whatever skills you find in your group, remember, there are many jobs to do, many ways to help, and all of them are important.

Preparing for Your Part of the Meeting

Now that you've thought about the people coming to the meeting in terms of what they may be able to contribute, you need to study the meeting itself. The leader will need to study the exercises for part one of the meeting, and the coordinator will need to study the exercises for part two.

The Leader

If you're the leader, you should familiarize yourself with exercises 1, 2, 3, 4, 10, and 11, and follow the step-by-step guide for each exercise. (You will find the detailed instructions and suggested scripts in chapters 7 and 8.)

THE EXERCISES—AN OVERVIEW

Here is an overview of the exercises you will lead and their purposes.

EXERCISE 1
Introductions

Purpose
- To introduce everyone to everyone
- To help everyone feel comfortable
- To learn the resources of the group

EXERCISE 2
The Person Who Is Ill Addresses the Group

Purpose
- To bring everyone up-to-date on the person's illness
- To give the person who is ill an opportunity to express his or her feelings
- To be sure the person who is ill is included in the meeting

EXERCISE 3
Feelings, Part One

Purpose
- To make it safe and easy for everyone to talk about their feelings

EXERCISE 4
Something for You

Purpose
- To make people in the group realize there can and will be hidden benefits to being a member
- To let the person who is ill know that the group isn't doing this just for him or her

EXERCISE 10
The Seven Principles

Purpose
- To introduce the Seven Principles in a fresh, interesting way
- To involve everyone in them
- To bond the group in another way

EXERCISE 11
Feelings, Part Two

Purpose
- To make it safe and easy for everyone to talk about their feelings
- To see how people are feeling after the meeting
- To see how feelings can change

As you study the exercises you will lead, make notes for yourself or use the suggested script if you feel more comfortable having something to follow.

Add some of your own words—make the script sound as if it came from you. Be sure to rehearse and work out the opening and closing with your co-ordinator. Perhaps you and the coordinator can help each other by following each other's scripts as you speak to make sure no important points are missed. Remember, you are a team helping to get a larger team on its feet.

The Coordinator

If you're the coordinator, you should familiarize yourself with exercises 5, 6, 7, 8, and 9, and follow the step-by-step guide for each exercise. (You will find the detailed instructions and suggested scripts in chapter 8.)

You will also download a set of forms and schedules for use in the meeting, following the guidelines and examples given in the Workbook (chapter 9).

THE EXERCISES—AN OVERVIEW

Here is an overview of the exercises you will lead and their purposes.

EXERCISE 5
Getting to Know All About You

Purpose
- To collect everyone's vital statistics and availabilities
- To take the first step toward commitment

Forms you will need*
- The Individual Data Form (blank form)

EXERCISE 6
Limits

Purpose
- To make sure the right people are doing the right jobs
- To keep people from promising more than they can do
- To give everyone permission to say no

---

* When you do the actual exercises in chapter 8, you will see samples of completed forms for your information. The blank master forms for photocopying are in chapter 9, and are also available online.

Forms you will need

- Your Limits, Strengths, and Weaknesses (blank forms)

EXERCISE 7
Captains

Purpose

- To make sure someone is always in charge
- To make sure no one is overburdened
- To keep the person who is ill from feeling guilty about asking for help all the time
- To help the person who is ill feel secure

Forms you will need

- The Rotating Captain's Schedule (filled-in sample form)
- The Caring Schedule (filled-in sample form)

EXERCISE 8
The Telephone Tree for Emergencies

Purpose

- To make sure all information gets to everyone quickly
- To make sure no one has to make more than two phone calls at any one time

Forms you will need

- The Telephone Tree (filled-in sample form)

EXERCISE 9
The Yellow Pages and the Group E-mail List

Purpose

- To have all necessary information in one place at one time
- To make it easier to handle an emergency

Forms you will need

- The Yellow Pages (filled-in sample forms)
- The Group E-mail List (filled-in sample form)

As you study the exercises you will lead, make notes for yourself to make the suggested scripts more comfortable and personal.

CHAPTER SEVEN

The Meeting, Part One: Getting to Know Each Other

Are You Ready?

Whether you are the leader or the coordinator, you're ready for your first meeting if:

- You have read and studied chapters 6, 7, 8, and 9.
- You have spoken personally to everyone who's coming.
- You have photocopied the set of forms from chapter 9.
- You have made name tags for everyone who's coming and put them in a place where they can be easily picked up when people enter the room.
- You have brought the refreshments and they are laid out and ready for your meeting break.
- You have made sure there will be no interruptions at the meeting.

If You Are Leading the Meeting

The first meeting is as much about sharing feelings as it is about ideas and exercises. If you are the leader, your purposes are to create an environment where everyone feels comfortable sharing feelings, to make sure everyone gets called on, and to listen to each person carefully, with no judgments about what he or she is saying. It is also important that you share your own feelings with the group and do each exercise as fully as everyone else. (You might want to do them first by yourself so they are familiar to you.)

If the person who is ill or his biological family or friends have been denying how sick he really is, this meeting may bring out their true fears. This is when you must trust the group. You do not have to deal with everything that comes up. Remember, everyone is afraid and no one has all the answers.

When people arrive, thank them for coming. Allow them a few minutes to mix and meet each other. *But keep track of the time.* The meeting is designed to last approximately three and a half hours (one and a half hours for part one, a fifteen- to twenty-minute refreshment break, and one and a half hours for part two). The time will differ depending upon how many people you have in the meeting and how willing they are to share with the group. Don't start more than fifteen minutes late. It is up to you to quiet the room, make sure everyone is comfortably seated, and begin the meeting.

Note to Leader: Using past meetings, we have suggested actual words or "scripts" you may want to use when conducting your first meeting. Study them and then, if you wish, use your own words. This is *your* group, and the more you are yourself, the more relaxed everyone will be.

Meeting Introduction

Suggested Script for Leader

Thank you for coming and welcome. And thank you [name of person whose home it is] for having us in your home. It is nice to see so many friends of [name of friend who is ill] here tonight.

Before we get started, please turn off your cell phones and pagers. There is a lot of information to cover, so we will follow a plan and [name of coordinator] and I will lead us through the evening. We will be doing several key exercises that all Share The Care groups have done.

This meeting will have two parts. In the first part we will lay the groundwork for how we can help [your friend] and each other, and in the second part, we will be setting up the practical systems and guidelines that make the group work.

I will take you through part one and [coordinator] will take you through part two. We will take a fifteen- to twenty-minute refreshment break in between. The meeting will last about three and a half hours.

The two main purposes of this group will be:

1. *To reduce all stress on [your friend] so he/she can concentrate on his/her mental and physical health;*
2. *To create an experience of helping him/her that is enlivening and nurturing for everyone in the group.*
   Let's begin with finding out who is here.

Note to Leader: If people want to ask questions, suggest they wait until part two of the meeting, when there will be time allowed.

EXERCISE 1
Introductions

Purpose
- To introduce everyone to everyone
- To help everyone feel comfortable
- To learn the resources of the group

Materials you will need
- Name tags, which you have prepared in advance

Time needed
- Two or three minutes per person

Note to Leader: Even if everyone in the room knows everyone else, it is still important to do this part. When everyone speaks, it sets the groundwork for later sharing. Asking them why they are here lets the person who is ill learn how her friends feel about being here. As everyone speaks, you may also discover things you didn't know about people you've been friends with for years. Make sure everyone is wearing a name tag. Also, make sure people say what they do for a living, because this will reveal the resources available to the group. Someone might have a computer, someone a car, someone might be in the medical profession or in insurance, someone might work in a grocery store, a drugstore, and so on. The section "Identifying Your Group's Skills" in chapter 6 will help you with this.

Suggested Script for Leader

Let's go around the room and introduce ourselves. Say your name, what you
do with your time, how you earn a living, and how you know [your friend].
Be sure to tell us how you came to be here tonight. Just take a minute or two.

EXERCISE 2
The Person Who Is Ill Addresses the Group

Purpose
- To bring everyone up-to-date on the person's illness
- To give the person who is ill an opportunity to express his or her feelings
- To be sure the person who is ill is included in the meeting

Materials you will need
- None

Time needed
- Approximately fifteen minutes

Note to Leader: It is important to let the person who needs help have a role
in the meeting. At this point, they will probably have heard their friends
express their love and they will want to talk. They will probably cry. Let
them. Don't interrupt. Give them time to express themselves fully. (You
may want to have a box of tissues in the room.) If they don't talk about
what they need or what they are afraid of, gently ask. They will probably
talk about how hard it is to ask for help and how guilty they feel asking all
these people. Reassure them again that the group is a way for them not to
have to ask all the time and not to feel guilty.

If you are the leader, be sure to call the person who is ill before the
meeting and tell him or her that you will be asking him or her to speak. If
the patient is very ill or tired, and the meeting is going to be held at the
patient's home, tell the ill person that he or she may go into another room
and lie down, especially during the second part of the meeting, which is
more about logistics. If the meeting is to be held at another person's
home, make arrangements for the patient to be able to lie down in another room if necessary.

Suggested Script for Leader

[Your friend], please tell the group what is going on. Tell us about your health, what the doctors say, how you feel. Also, tell us what you need and what you are most afraid of.

EXERCISE 3
Feelings, Part One

Purpose
- To make it safe and easy for everyone to talk about their feelings

Materials you will need
- A bowl
- One index card (blank on both sides) for each person in attendance
- Pencils

Time needed
- Approximately twenty minutes

Note to Leader: In this exercise, people write what they are feeling on cards. The cards are put in a bowl, mixed up, and everyone draws someone else's card and reads it out loud. The purpose of this exercise is to show us that we all share the same fears, feelings, and thoughts. No matter which card a person draws, it will probably apply to that person to some degree or other. Hearing all the sentences will allow everyone to get in touch with and share their feelings safely without having to state them as their own. Do not call on people to read. Let them read their card when they feel ready. Make sure people do not rush this exercise, but make sure everyone reads a card.

Suggested Script for Leader

Please take a card. Be sure not to put your name on it.

Please print this sentence and then complete it: "What I am feeling right now is   ."

Take your time. When you are finished, fold your card so the writing doesn't show and place your card in the bowl.

Note to Leader: Make sure everyone puts their card into the bowl. Make sure each card is folded so the writing cannot be seen. Mix up the cards. Pass the bowl around.

Suggested Script for Leader

Please select a folded card.

This is now your card. Take a moment to read silently what is written on your card.

Make believe that you have written what is on the card. Take a minute and feel what the words say. If it is, in fact, your card, don't tell us.

When you are ready, read the card you selected to us as if it were your own.

If you have received a blank card, make up the sentence.

Note to Leader: Here are examples of the kinds of things that may be written:

What I am feeling right now is "helpless."

What I am feeling right now is "I wish I could take this illness away from [your friend]."

What I am feeling right now is "very worried."

EXERCISE 4
Something for You

Purpose

- To make people in the group realize there can and will be hidden benefits to being a member
- To let the person who is ill know that the group isn't doing this just for him or her

Materials you will need

- Pencils and pads

Time needed

- Approximately twenty minutes

Note to Leader: This can be the most difficult exercise you will have to do with your group. People may not understand what you mean, or they may feel guilty about admitting they can get something for themselves. But insist that they write something and encourage them to be honest. It is very important that people give a personal answer.

Give everyone enough time to think about this and write down an answer. When all, or everyone but one or two people, are finished, ask everyone to share what they have written.

The best way to help people with a difficult exercise such as this one is to "model" it. As leader, you serve as the model and state what you think you can gain personally from being in the group. For your use, here are some examples of what people have said in previous meetings. We do not suggest sharing them with the group unless everyone is confused by the question and reticent about sharing.

> *"I feel that a support group such as this one will help me keep my own everyday problems in perspective."*

> *"I want to feel like I know how to take care of someone, and that I am a capable, responsible woman. I also need to know I can be a friend through and through, . . . go all the way . . . to the wire. No matter what."*

> *"Before my father was in the nursing home, I had been taking care of him all by myself for years and I know how hard it is to be the only one. I think it will be wonderful not having to do this all by myself."*

Suggested Script for Leader

A caregiver group won't work unless everyone gets something out of it personally. So I want you to think about some things you might get just for your-

self by being a member of the group, something that has nothing to do with [your friend], and write them down. Think of things that will benefit you.

This exercise forms one of the key foundation blocks of every group. If we are not getting something for ourselves, [your friend] will feel too guilty. Also, to stay in this group, we may have to draw on deep inner reserves. It will help us to do this later if we are clear now that we are getting something for ourselves out of being in the group.

Note to Leader: After this exercise, ask [your friend] if he or she has anything to say. He or she will probably be relieved to realize that the members of the group have something to gain just for themselves.

Part One: Conclusion

Suggested Script for Leader

This concludes part one of our meeting. We are now going to take a short refreshment break. We have sandwiches, cookies, and soft drinks for everyone. We will start part two of the meeting at [note time and allow fifteen to twenty minutes].

Note to Leader: Take a refreshment break for fifteen to twenty minutes. During the break, talk to the person who is ill. See how he or she is holding up. Encourage the person to stay for the second part of the meeting, but if he or she is very tired or feeling poorly, allow him or her to leave or go into the next room and lie down.

Note to Leader and Coordinator: If you followed the previous chapter and did part one of your meeting carefully, your group will be well on its way to becoming a Share The Care family.

As people expressed their feelings, the person who is ill was probably very comforted by all the love in the room. Everyone, in fact, was probably moved by the group's sincere desire to help someone in need and by the realization that this may prove to be a very meaningful experience for them. As each person discovered what he or she might gain from being part of the group, all are now probably more comfortable about committing to it.

Now it's time to get to work and put *your* unique group into operation.

What is part two of your meeting about?

In part two, you will focus on the practical systems and principles that make the group run. The exercises in chapter 8 are keyed to filled-in samples of the forms and schedules in chapter 9. (If you are reading this for the first time, before the meeting, you might want to skip ahead to chapter 9 and familiarize yourself with the forms and explanations given there.)

But part two of the meeting is more than practical advice. It also has its emotional challenges. The person who is ill will have to give up some control in order to get the help he or she needs. The group will be confronted with issues of commitment, limits, and control. These things are not easy for most of us. Most group members will be experiencing feelings that are not necessarily part of their everyday lives. Many will be facing issues and feelings they would rather not express.

CHAPTER EIGHT

The Meeting, Part Two: Getting Organized

Note to Leader: If you are the leader of part two of the meeting, your job is to help group members get clear about what they are willing to do and what they are not willing to do. You must also help them to be clear about what they are good at and not so good at. One or two people have probably been trying to do all the work involved with helping someone who is ill. They may have become very attached to being so needed, even if they're exhausted. You need to continually reinforce the idea of the power of the group and make sure everyone sticks to the exercises and the format.

You will probably also have to help the person who is ill to let go, to stop trying to run everything, and to let other people do things he or she has been trying to do alone. It may not be easy for people who are ill to let all these other people into their lives. Remember, until you made these phone calls, they were running the show, doing the best they could. You need to be patient and understanding, yet firm, and never forget that the person who is ill is not just an illness but a complex, feeling human being.

Note to Coordinator: If you are the coordinator of part two of the meeting, your job is to get the group running. This means putting several systems into place, explaining the various forms and schedules, and coordinating *everything*. Remember, if you expect a large turnout, enlist an assistant to help you prepare. (See chapter 9, "Checklist for the Coordinator," p. 118.)

But you have another responsibility. It is your job to simplify the paperwork and systems for everyone else. You can do this only if you have taken the time beforehand to understand and be comfortable with all the information in chapter 9. You may find it necessary to tailor some of the forms to the needs of the person who is ill. For example, if your friend is about to face a difficult week, you need to make sure that the Caring Schedule for that week is set up before the meeting ends.

The Meeting, Part Two: Introduction

Suggested Script for Leader

Is everyone comfortable and ready to begin? Are all cell phones off?

This second part of the meeting is about how we can make helping [your friend] a positive, nurturing experience for us all without any one person's feeling overburdened. It is also about [your friend's] willingness to let us help.

There are several principles and systems Share The Care has discovered that all groups use and find important. [Name of coordinator] will be handing out worksheets, schedules, and forms that will, in effect, put our caregiver group into operation tonight.

Note to Coordinator: To run this next part of the meeting, you will need to have studied part 3 (chapters 10 through 18): "Being Part of a Group and Sharing the Jobs," especially the list of jobs on pages 154 through 155. You can read from it to get people thinking. Or better yet, make a list of jobs you know will be needed right away.

Suggested Script for Coordinator

Hi, I'm [coordinator], and I'm going to be our coordinator. I'm here to get us organized and keep us going as a group.

But before we get to the paperwork and the systems, let's talk about what it is that members do.

- *Errands and housekeeping*
  We help [your friend] do all the errands that are hard to keep up with even when we're well. Errands such as grocery shopping, run-

ning to the pharmacy, going to the dry cleaner, and doing the laundry. We also help [your friend] around the house. We do the cooking, vacuuming, straightening up. We will be setting up a system tonight to make it easier to do these errands.

- **Special tasks**

    Just when you need to be doing less, there are all the extra things you are faced with when you have a serious illness. For example, picking up X-rays from one doctor and delivering them to another, making doctors' appointments, arranging hospital admittance or finding a physical therapist, picking up books or researching information on the Internet. We will be setting up a system tonight that will make it easier to do these tasks.

- **Serving as companions**

    Other groups have found that one of the most important things we can do is accompany [your friend] to doctors, radiation appointments, hospitals, medical centers for tests or therapy, or, for that matter, out to dinner or the movies. We can be there the night before surgery or when [your friend] comes back from recovery. We can simply keep [your friend] company in waiting rooms, hail taxis in the rain, try to decipher what doctors are saying. We can be his/her ears, listen and write things down, help formulate questions before a key appointment. Even the smallest thing can make a huge difference when you're tired, scared, or in pain.

- **Being there for one another**

    Sometimes, another member may need you as much as the person who is ill. We may need one another to solve a problem, make a decision, or just hang out. The one thing every group member needs to realize is "Don't try to do it alone." As of tonight, we don't have to. The general rule is "If it's easy, one person goes. If it's difficult, send two people. If it's very difficult, three." When in doubt, always take an extra person. So one of us can just be with [your friend] while another handles logistics. Or one of us can just be with [your friend], one can handle logistics, and the third can get lunch and calm the nerves of the other two.

Now, how do we get all this done? We follow the Share The Care system! As the meeting goes on, I'll be asking you to fill out some forms and answer some questions. After the meeting, I will collect and coordinate all the information. In about a week, I will mail each of you a set of everything you need. I hope to make being a part of this group easy and to keep you all from drowning in paperwork. The first form we will be using is the three-page Individual Data Form.

Note to Coordinator: Pass out Individual Data Forms to be filled out. (Blank forms can be downloaded and edited from the Web site, http://www .sharethecare.org; or are available for photocopying on pages 103–105.) For your convenience, completed sample forms follow the exercises so you don't have to skip ahead to chapter 9, The Workbook. The completed Individual Data Form sample can be found on pages 79 to 81.

EXERCISE 5
Getting to Know All About You

Purpose
- To collect everyone's vital statistics and availabilities
- To take the first step toward commitment

Forms you will need
- Blank Individual Data Forms (page 1 only for this exercise) for each person to fill out (see chapter 9, page 103).

Time needed
- Fifteen minutes

Note to Coordinator: This is the point in the meeting where each person will begin to get an idea of the commitment required to be part of the group. Give them permission to say no. Encourage them to say what they are afraid of, what they are hopeless at, and to be truthful about their abilities, their dislikes, and their strengths. When they have finished, ask for volunteers to share what they have written as their strengths and weaknesses. There may be talking and joking within the group with this exercise. Don't rush. Enjoy it!

Suggested Script for Coordinator

The first page of the Individual Data Form will give the group easy access to everyone's vital statistics and availabilities. During the life of our group, everyone will probably need to know how and when to contact everyone else in the group. These pages will be used as part of a "captain" system that we will be setting up and ultimately will be part of the Yellow Pages and the Group E-mail List that I will be assembling later. Take a minute to fill them out now.

It is important for us to recognize that we are about to make a real commitment and to take the time to look and see if we can commit to being in the group and how much of a commitment we can make.

Really think about your availability. What days of the week are best for you? What times of day are best for you?

Can you commit to being a full member or do you want to be a free-floater? A free-floater is someone who fills in when regular members are not available and is also an important part of making the group work. It's okay if that is all you feel you can do.

Now turn to pages 2 and 3 of your Individual Data Form. This part is called "Your Limits, Strengths, and Weaknesses."

Note to Coordinator: Check to see that everyone has completed the first page. If they haven't, ask how much more time they need. Proceed when everyone or almost everyone has completed page 1.

EXERCISE 6
Limits

Purpose
- To make sure the right people are doing the right jobs
- To keep people from promising more than they can do
- To give everyone permission to say no

Forms you will need
- Blank pages 2 and 3 of the Individual Data Form—Your Limits, Strengths, and Weaknesses—for each person to fill out (see chapter 9, pages 104 and 105).

Time needed

- Twenty minutes

Suggested Script for Coordinator

The first key to making sure no one member of the group burns out is being clear about our strengths and weaknesses. As the saying goes, "If we can't trust your no, we can't trust your yes." This form is designed to find the right person for the right job whenever possible. Look at the second page of the Individual Data Form and consider the list carefully. As you check the boxes, be honest.

- *How are you in emergencies?*
- *Can you handle a lot of information at once?*
- *Does paperwork make you dizzy?*
- *Does the sight of blood make you pass out?*
- *Can you talk to doctors?*
- *Are you good at remembering names? Details?*

Note to Coordinator: For your convenience, there is a blank copy of "Your Limits, Strengths, and Weaknesses" available on the Web site. This will allow you to download. Fill in the specific types of skills you need to find or the jobs you need to fill.

Now turn to the third page. We've given you space to tell us anything we may have left out. Remember, everyone has limits. One of the most important principles of a successful caregiver group is understanding what our limits are. No one has to do everything. Things one person fears, hates, or is not good at, another person may be able to do easily.

Note to Coordinator: Collect all sheets. Make sure everyone's questions have been answered before moving on.

Note to <u>COORDINATOR</u>:
- Use in first meeting.
- Copy on blue-tinted paper
- Staple together with pages 2, 3.

Date: **4/02/04**

SHARE THE CARE

INDIVIDUAL DATA FORM

(page 1)

Name **Jackie G.**

Address: Street **121 Cherry Hill Road**   Apt. **12B**

City **NY**   State **NY**   Zip **10000**

Home phone: (212) 555-1111

Work phone: (212) 555-1212

Other phone: (weekend home) (314) 555-1010

Fax: (212) 555-0000

Cell: (212) 555-9999

E-mail: jackieg@example.com

Occupation: **parttime graphic designer/Yoga Instructor**

Do you have a car?   yes ( )   no (✔) If not, can you drive?   yes (✔)   no ( )

Can you participate as a Share The Care member?   yes (✔)   no ( )

If you feel you cannot participate as a Share The Care member,
can you commit to being a free-floater?   yes ( )   no ( )

AVAILABILITY: Are there any days or specific hours when you know you would <u>not be</u>
<u>available?</u> Please indicate in the chart below:

Time	Monday	Tuesday	Wednesday	Thursday	Friday	Saturday	Sunday
9:00 A.M. 1:00 P.M.						*(JUNE-SEPT)*	
1:00 P.M. 5:00 P.M.						*In summer I try to get out of town to beach every other weekend—but I can be flexible.*	
5:00 P.M. 10:00 P.M.	*June-July 6-9:00 (Seminar)*		*Every Weds. 7-10 PM PHOTOG. CLASS*				
10:00 P.M. Overnight							

OTHER: (Specific dates) **June 25-27 out of town (wedding)**

Sept. 6-12 vacation (beach)

NOTE TO <u>COORDINATOR</u>:
• Use in first meeting.
• Copy on blue-tinted paper.
• Staple together with pages 1, 3.

Date: __4/02/04__

INDIVIDUAL DATA FORM
YOUR LIMITS, STRENGTHS, AND WEAKNESSES

(page 2)

Name   *Jackie G.*

This form is designed to try to find the right person for the job whenever possible.

Where do you fit in when it comes to the following areas?

Remember, it's okay not to like something or not to be good at another thing. Someone else in the group may like to do what you don't. Rate yourself on the following:

IN DEALING WITH	I'M TERRIFIC	I'M GOOD	I'M FAIR	DON'T CALL ON ME
Emergencies	✔			
Paperwork organization		✔		
Insurance forms		✔		
Hospitals	✔			
Talking to doctors	✔			
Physical tasks	✔			
Cooking special foods	✔			
Research		✔		
Xeroxing paperwork	✔			
Listening and taking notes		✔		
Asking questions		✔		
Needles		✔		
Blood		✔		
Making appointments		✔		
Shopping (grocery)	✔			
Shopping (personal items)			✔	
Hiring help			✔	
Firing help				✔
Housecleaning				✔
Finding solutions to problems	✔			

NOTE TO <u>COORDINATOR</u>:
- Use in first meeting.
- Copy on blue-tinted paper.
- Staple together with pages 1, 2.

Date: __4/02/04__

INDIVIDUAL DATA FORM
YOUR LIMITS, STRENGTHS, AND WEAKNESSES

(page 3)

Name ___Jackie G.___

In your own words, is there anything else that you want to tell us about
what you like to do, are a "star" at doing, don't want to do, or abhor?

I am truly great at:

Basically I have a calming personality so I'm good when others get nervous.

I'm good at finding solutions and getting things organized.

I have some caregiving experience - my aunt broke her hip and needed my help

for several months.

My schedule is always changing - I have some free time during the middle of the

day.

I absolutely cannot deal with:

I hate doing laundry and cleaning.

Special skills and hobbies: *I have CPR training, and excellent computer skills,*

love to cook, photography, and am a Yoga Instructor.

<u>*Maybe I could help with physical therapy exercises!!*</u>

EXERCISE 7

Captains

Purpose

- To make sure someone is always in charge
- To make sure no one is overburdened
- To keep the person who is ill from feeling guilty about asking for help all the time
- To help the person who is ill feel secure

Forms you will need

- The Rotating Captain's Schedule—completed sample for each person. (See page 85. When photocopying, enlarge to 150%.)
- The Caring Schedule—completed sample for each person (see page 86).

Time needed

- Fifteen minutes

Note to Coordinator: You may run into several kinds of opposition to the captain system. The person who is sick has probably been relying heavily on one or two people and, while these people may be burning out, both they and the person who is ill may believe they are the only people who can help. You must make it clear that the person who is ill is not losing this closeness but will actually have more quality time with this friend or parent or daughter because the caregiver will not be so overburdened.

Be sure to stress that the captain system keeps the person who is ill from having to constantly ask for help. Remember, every time the patient has to ask, he or she is reminded of frailty, limits, and an increasing loss of control. Such people feel guilty that they're ruining their friends' or family's lives, angry that they can no longer do things for themselves, and frightened that things will not be taken care of.

Suggested Script for Coordinator

The second key to making the group work is sharing responsibility. No one person has to be in charge or on call all the time. No one person has to deal with every problem or emergency. *Everyone has something special to contribute. There is no one "right way" to do anything.* To ensure that no one will be overburdened, we're going to set up the captain system.

Being captain is the most important job you will have as a member.

What Is the Captain System?

The captain system assures that someone will always be in charge and that no one has to be in charge all the time. Captains work in pairs, and two captains (co-captains) are assigned to work together overseeing everything for one week at a time. As co-captains, you can divide the duties equally, do difficult tasks together, or substitute for each other if one of you has a personal emergency or is unable to do her or his part. So if there are twelve of you, you will each be a co-captain only once every six weeks.

What Do Captains Do?

The captains are in charge of scheduling everything for their week. How do they do this? They follow a simple step-by-step process.

- *Talk to the person who is ill or their family and find out what will be needed that week.*
- *Prioritize the jobs.*
- *Consult the Individual Data Sheet for abilities and availabilities of members.*
- *Call and/or e-mail members and schedule the various jobs.*
- *Fill in the schedule.*
- *Give a copy to the person who is ill so he or she will know who will be doing what.*

The captains are responsible for getting information out, contacting doctors, and making sure medicine is picked up, dinners are provided, and errands are run. They are also responsible for handling any crises that arise during their week.

Why the Captain System Is Critical for Members

- *On the weeks we're not captain, we don't have to think about anything except what we're individually scheduled for.*

- *We always have a co-captain, so if we have a crisis in our own life, our partner can take over.*
- *We always have someone to talk to, complain to, acknowledge us, or hold our hand.*

Why the Captain System Is Critical for the People Who Are Ill

- *They only have to talk to one captain every week, so they don't feel as if they're asking for help all the time.*
- *They can rest easy, knowing that everything is being handled and no one is doing too much.*
- *They don't have to worry about any scheduling or paperwork themselves.*

Now I'm going to pass out two sample forms: The Rotating Captain's Schedule and the Caring Schedule. They're just examples to help you get the idea.

Note to Coordinator: Pass out copies of the completed samples of the Rotating Captain's Schedule and the Caring Schedule.

The Caring Schedule is a simple calendar for scheduling everything that will be needed for the week. As a captain, you will use it to fit members into specific needed time slots. You will also give a copy of the completed schedule to [your friend] so he will know whom to expect and when to expect them. This relieves any anxieties he might have about the upcoming week.

I will be sending you blank copies with your information packet.

Are there any two people who want to volunteer to be the first co-captains? Perhaps some of you want to pair up now and put your names on the list. If not, I will assign co-captains and make out a schedule for the next several months.

Remember, if you feel that you can't be a captain, but still want to help, you can still be in the group by being a free-floater. Not everyone has to be a captain. It is better to commit to what you can really do than to overcommit and not come through.

NOTE TO <u>COORDINATOR</u>: This schedule can be filled in, saved, and edited online, then printed. Copy on pink-tinted paper.	**SHARE THE CARE**	Date: __4/05/04__

ROTATING CAPTAIN'S SCHEDULE

A Share The Care week is: Monday, Tuesday, Wednesday, Thursday, Friday, Saturday, through and including Sunday.

IMPORTANT: If you absolutely cannot be captain for a specific week you must
1. Notify your co-captain.
2. Find a replacement, *and*
3. Let the group know via e-mail or telephone tree.

CAPTAINS	DATES (FOR WEEKS OF:)
1. Jackie G.	4/5 - 4/11, 5/24 - 5/30,
2. Beth R.	7/12 - 7/18, 8/30 - 9/5
1. Jane R.	4/12 - 4/18, 5/31 - 6/6
2. Donna D.	7/19 - 7/25, 9/6 - 9/12
1. Sharon A.	4/19 - 4/25, 6/7 - 6/13,
2. Cecelia T.	7/26 - 8/1, 9/13 — 9/19
1. Karen S.	4/26 - 5/2, 6/14 - 6/20,
2. Lee W.	8/2 - 8/8, 9/20 - 9/26
1. Brenda R.	5/3 - 5/9, 6/21 - 6/27,
2. Bill M.	8/9 - 8/15, 9/27 - 10/3
1. Bob C.	5/10 - 5/16, 6/28 - 7/4,
2. Julie K.	8/16 - 8/22, 10/4 - 10/10
1. Mark T.	5/17 - 5/23, 7/5 - 7/11,
2. Mary T.	8/23 - 8/29, 10/11 - 10/17

NOTE TO COORDINATOR:
Copy on pink-tinted paper.
Name: York Hospital
Address: 425 East 44th Street
(between 1st and York Aves.)
Room: 727   Tel: 212-555-8000 x727
Visiting Hrs: 12:00-8:00 PM

Dates: 5/24-5/30
Captain: Jackie G.
Captain: Beth R.

SHARE THE CARE
CARING SCHEDULE

DATES / TIME	MONDAY 5/24	TUESDAY 5/25	WEDNESDAY 5/26	THURSDAY 5/27	FRIDAY 5/28	SATURDAY 5/29	SUNDAY 5/30
9:00 A.M. / 1:00 P.M.	DR. APPT. Dr. Arnold T. (see yellow pgs) DONNA 10:30AM	*Hospital Check-in Jackie	Operation 8:00AM	No Visitors Til Noon	*Hospital Check-out 9:00AM Donna Brenda	Jane	Lisa Leslie (daughter)
1:00 P.M. / 5:00 P.M.	→ Lee Arr. 3:00PM		Hospital Visit Beth	Hospital Visit Bill	→	JOAN Arr. 1:30 Lisa (due in at 4:00PM) (daughter)	→
5:00 P.M. / 10:00 P.M.	→ Dinner Lee	Hospital Visit Jane	Hospital Visit Sharon	Hospital Visit Brenda	Dinner Beth Arr By 5:00	Dinner Cecelia Lisa	Dinner JOAN
Overnight	Overnight Jackie Arr. 7:00PM	Hosp.	Hosp.	Hosp.	Overnight Jane Arr. 7:30PM	Overnight Lisa	Overnight Karen Arr. 6:00PM Lisa, Leslie back to school

EXERCISE 8

The Telephone Tree for Emergencies

Purpose

- To make sure all urgent information gets to everyone quickly
- To make sure that no one has to make more than two phone calls at any one time

Materials you will need

- The Telephone Tree—completed sample for each person (see page 88)

Time needed

- Ten minutes

Note to Coordinator: Pass out the example of a Telephone Tree.

Suggested Script for Coordinator

The Telephone Tree is the fastest way to reach everyone in the group in case of an emergency. It is a simple way to make sure no one has to make more than two telephone calls.

This is an example of a Telephone Tree. You will be getting a real one for our group in your information packet. The Telephone Tree contains all telephone numbers where members can be reached at any time: home, work, cell phones, weekend home, and any other number that is not included in the sample.

I will put[your friend]'s name at the top of the tree followed by Position A, the person with the most daily contact.

- *If you have information to pass along the tree, contact the person in Position A, then call the person directly under you.*
- *Each person is responsible for getting information down the tree.*
- *If you cannot reach the person directly under you, call the next person down on the tree. Then be sure to go back later and call the person you missed.*
- *If you have to leave a message on voice mail, also call the next person down on the tree (the first person could be out of town).*

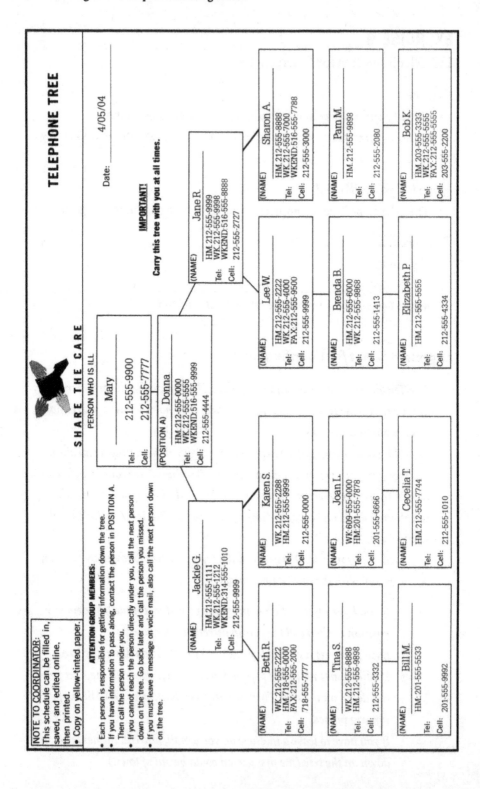

TELEPHONE TREE

Date: _____ 4/05/04

IMPORTANT!
Carry this tree with you at all times.

SHARE THE CARE

PERSON WHO IS ILL

Mary
Tel: 212-555-9900
Cell: 212-555-7777

NOTE TO COORDINATOR:
This schedule can be filled in,
saved, and edited online,
then printed.
• Copy on yellow-tinted paper.

ATTENTION GROUP MEMBERS:

• Each person is responsible for getting information down the tree.
• If you have information to pass along, contact the person in POSITION A.
  Then call the person under you.
• If you cannot reach the person directly under you, call the next person
  down on the tree. Go back later and call the person you missed.
• If you must leave a message on voice mail, also call the next person down
  on the tree.

(POSITION A) Donna
HM.212-555-0000
WK.212-555-5555
WKEND.516-555-9999
Tel:
Cell: 212-555-4444

(NAME) Jane R.
HM.212-555-9999
WK.212-555-9998
WKEND.516-555-8888
Tel:
Cell: 212-555-2727

(NAME) Jackie G.
HM.212-555-1111
WK.212-555-1212
WKEND.314-555-1010
Tel:
Cell: 212-555-9999

(NAME) Karen S.
WK.212-555-2288
HM.212-555-9999
Tel:
Cell: 212-555-0000

(NAME) Lee W.
HM.212-555-2222
WK.212-555-4000
FAX.212-555-9500
Tel:
Cell: 212-555-9999

(NAME) Sharon A.
HM.212-555-8888
WK.212-555-7000
WKEND.516-555-7788
Tel:
Cell: 212-555-3000

(NAME) Beth R.
WK.212-555-2222
HM.718-555-0000
FAX.212-555-2000
Tel:
Cell: 718-555-7777

(NAME) Joan L.
WK.609-555-0000
HM.201-555-7878
Tel:
Cell: 201-555-6666

(NAME) Brenda B.
HM.212-555-6000
WK.212-555-9868
Tel:
Cell: 212-555-1413

(NAME) Pam M.
HM.212-555-9898
Tel:
Cell: 212-555-2080

(NAME) Tina S
WK.212-555-8888
HM.212-555-9898
Tel:
Cell: 212-555-3332

(NAME) Cecelia T
HM.212-555-7744
Tel:
Cell: 212-555-1010

(NAME) Elizabeth P
HM.212-555-5555
Tel:
Cell: 212-555-4334

(NAME) Bob K.
HM.203-555-3333
WK.212-555-5555
FAX.212-555-5555
Tel:
Cell: 203-555-2200

(NAME) Bill M.
HM.201-555-5533
Tel:
Cell: 201-555-9992

- *Carry your copy of this tree with you at all times. Keep an extra copy in your weekend home, office, or car.*

You will use your Telephone Tree whenever you need to contact all the members; for example, you would use it in these situations:

- *The person who is ill has been admitted to the hospital due to an emergency*
- *The person who is ill does not want to be disturbed by phone calls*
- *The group suddenly needs to call a meeting*

Are there any questions?

EXERCISE 9

The Yellow Pages and the Group E-mail List

Purpose
- To have all necessary information in one place at one time
- To make it easier to handle an emergency

Materials you will need
- The Yellow Pages—completed sample for each person (see pages 91 to 95)

Time Needed
- Ten minutes

Note to Coordinator: Pass out sample copies of Yellow Pages.

Suggested Script for Coordinator

This is an example of the Yellow Pages. As you can see, it contains all the names and numbers of anyone you might need in order to help the person who is ill at any time of the day or night.

- *Group members*
- *Real family members*
- *Free-floaters*

- *Babysitters, landlord, super, handyman, cleaning lady*
- *Doctors, therapists, surgeons, technicians (including names of their respective nurses, secretaries, and receptionists)*
- *Pharmacy: include name of pharmacist (special instructions)*
- *Medical insurance information: name of advocate, group insurance numbers, Social Security number for person who is ill*

I will be sending you each a copy of our Yellow Pages in your information packet when I have coordinated all the information needed.

You should all carry your Yellow Pages (along with a copy of the Telephone Tree) at all times. If you have a weekend home, an office, or a car, it is also a good idea to leave an extra copy there.

Copies of the Yellow Pages should also be kept in a designated place by each of the telephones at the home of the person who is ill.

You will also receive a hard copy of the Group E-mail List. Please enter all the names into your computer as a group for your convenience. If any of you don't have a computer or access to e-mail, please let me know. We will make arrangements for someone to contact you by phone with important information, since we will be doing a good deal of communicating through e-mail in order to save time.

Now I'm going to turn the meeting over to [name of leader] for our last two exercises.

Note to Coordinator: Be sure to list the names of people with no e-mail. Once you find out who they are, get volunteers or ask someone to call those people with the messages they miss on group e-mail. Encourage members without e-mail to get it as soon as possible and to check it at least twice a day.

EXERCISE 10
The Seven Principles

Purpose
- To introduce the Seven Principles in a fresh, interesting way
- To involve everyone in them
- To bond the group in another way

NOTE TO COORDINATOR: This form can be filled in, saved, and edited online, then printed. • Copy on yellow-tinted paper. • Staple together pages 1–5.			Date: 4/05/04

SHARE THE CARE
YELLOW PAGES

CAREGIVER GROUP MEMBERS		(INCLUDE AREA CODE)	
NAME & ADDRESS	**TELEPHONE**	**CELL NUMBER**	**E-MAIL**
Jackie G. 121 Cherry Hill Road New York, N.Y. 10000 fax: 212-555-0000	home 212-555-1111 work 212-555-1212 wkend. 314-555-1010	212-555-9999	jackieg@example.com
Jane R. 337 East Choctaw Lane #6-A New York, N.Y. 10000 fax: 212-555-9900 (at work)	home 212-555-9999 work 212-555-9998 wkend 516-555-8888	212-555-2727	JaneR@example.com
Donna D. 55 East Fern Drive 3F New York, N.Y. 10000 fax: 212-555-0000	home 212-555-0000 work 212-555-5555 wkend 516-555-9999	212-555-4444	Donagirl@for.example.net
Beth R. 715 Grover Grange #4 Brooklyn, N.Y. 10000 fax:718-555-2000	home 718-555-0000 work 212-555-2222	718-555-7777	atbeach@example.net
Karen S. 55 West Pilgrims Pass 1209 New York, N.Y. 10000	home 212-555-9999 work 212-555-2288	212-555-0000	Art&art@example.org
Lee W. 123 West Rose Street 12F New York, N.Y. 10000 fax: 212-555-9900 (work)	home 212-555-2222 work 212-555-0000	212-555-9999	Whitlaw@for.example.net
Sharon A. 33 East Minske Meadows 3C New York, N.Y. 10000	home 212-555-8888 work 212-555-7000 wkend. 516-555-7788	212-555-3000	Sharon33@example.net

P. 2 — Copy on yellow-tinted paper.			Date: 4/05/04
REAL FAMILY	(INCLUDE AREA CODE)		
NAME & ADDRESS	**TELEPHONE**	**CELL NUMBER**	**E-MAIL**
Lisa T. (daughter) 767-Woodbury Road 3B Kenosha, WI 30000	hm. 508-555-8888	508-555-2222	Lisat@for.example.com
Leslie T. (daughter) Box 34 New Haven College New Haven, CT 20000	hm. 203-555-6565	203-555-9898	Starlt@example.com
Mr. and Mrs. R. (parents) 454 Elm Street Ft. Lauderdale, FL 50000	hm. 309-555-9765	309-555-3333	homestead@example .org
James T. (ex-husband) 339 Chester Lane 12-D Half Moon Bay, CA 90000	hm. 313-555-0000 wk. 313-555-9977 fax. 313-555-4444	313-555-8787	James@business .example
Barbara S. (sister) 383 Goat Lane Miami, FL 50000	hm. 309-555-9898 wk. 309-555-2222	309-555-7777	barbaraone@ example.com

P. 3 — Copy on yellow-tinted paper.   Date: <u>4/05/04</u>

FREE-FLOATERS (INCLUDE AREA CODE)

NAME & ADDRESS	TELEPHONE	CELL NUMBER	E-MAIL
Tina S. (Cousin) Rosewood Lane #44 East Hill, N.J. 10000	hm. 201-555-4443	201-555-1212	Tsims@example.com
Elizabeth P 550 East Kepler Kill Lane (4G) New York, N.Y. 10000	hm 212-555-5555 wk. 212-555-4433	212-555-2344	Lizjoe@for.example.net
Bob K. 54 West Farm Road Westport, CT 20000	hm. 203-555-3333 wk. 212-555-9999	203-555-2334	bob@example.org
Pam M. 33 Winsome Mews (5F) New York, N.Y. 10000	hm. 212-555-1112 wk. 212-555-2110	212-555-8877	pmroads@example.net

OTHER (SUPERINTENDENT, BABYSITTER, HANDYMAN, LANDLORD)

NAME & ADDRESS	TELEPHONE	CELL NUMBER	E-MAIL
Kara R. (housecleaning lady)	hm. 718-555-4545	718-555-2222	house@example.org
Robert R. (superintendent)	hm. 212-555-2224 wk. 212-555-4455	212-555-3434 beeper 212-555-5533	robert430@example .com
Steve S. (repairman—all kinds of jobs)	hm. 212-555-8000 wk. 212-555-9900	212-555-2232	starman@for.example

P. 4 — Copy on yellow-tinted paper.			Date: 4/05/04
MEDICAL (INCLUDE NAME OF NURSE, RECEPTIONIST, SECRETARY)			(INCLUDE AREA CODE)
DOCTOR'S NAME & ADDRESS (include specialty)		**E-MAIL**	**TELEPHONE**
Dr. Harris H. 309 West Frank Street (4H) New York, N.Y. 10000	psychotherapist		212-555-7676
Dr Robert S. 430 West Advent Street (4B) New York, N.Y. 10000 Receptionist: Susan Nurse: Beth	oncologist		212-555-6000
Dr. Aaron Z. 54 East Advent Street L-A New York, N.Y. 10000 Receptionist: Karen Nurse: Linda	orthopedic surgeon		212-555-7654
Dr. Steven V. Hoover Hospital Building A, Room 12-B 1200 West Carter Avenue New York, N.Y. 10000 Mrs. Joanne S. (technician for Dr. V)	radiologist		212-555-7645
Dr. Martin M. 230 West Road Forest Hills, N.Y. 10000 Receptionist: Mellinda	holistic doctor		718-555-3333
Dr. Arnold T. 40 East Blue Lane (L-8) New York, N.Y. 10000 Nurse: Martha	surgeon		212-555-8800
Dr. Richard G. 44 West Rue Boulevard (4J) New York, N.Y. 10000	holistic consultant		212-555-9999
Katherine F. All-Care Nursing Services Speak to Kate	home health-care aide		212-555-2222 cell: 212-555-9090
Margaret L.	private-duty nurse		212-555-2311

P. 5 — Copy on yellow-tinted paper.		Date: 04/05/04

PHARMACY (INCLUDE NAME OF PHARMACIST)		(INCLUDE AREA CODE)
NAME & ADDRESS	**TELEPHONE**	**FAX AND E-MAIL**
Kane Pharmacy (prescriptions on file) 330 Rex Road New York, N.Y. 10000 Pharmacist: Fred S. or Bob K.	212-555-9606/7	same as tel.
Treetop Pharmacy 88 East Linda Lane New York, N.Y. 10000 Pharmacist: Sidney	212-555-7777	212-555-7778

MEDICAL INSURANCE		(INCLUDE AREA CODE)
NAME & ADDRESS	**TELEPHONE**	**FAX AND E-MAIL**
Nationwide Insurance P.O. Box 333 Notown, N.Y. 10000 Advocate: Mary J. or Madeline S.	203-555-9111 1-800-555-9855	203-555-9122
Claims Dept: I.D. Reade Companies Social Security # 078-05-1120 Group Insurance #332-909 Other Insurance: None Group members in charge of dealing with Insurance matters are Karen S. and Beth R.		

*Be sure to Include
Name of insurance
Group insurance number
Social Security Number
Any other specific company identification

```
                    Share The Care
                  Group E-Mail List
                   Date: 04/05/04

     Jackie G.       jackieg@example.com

     Jane R.         JaneR@example.com

     Donna D.        Donagirl@for.example.net

     Beth R.         atbeach@example.net

     Karen S.        Art&art@example.org

     Lee W.          Whitlaw@for.example

     Sharon A.       Sharon33@example.net

     Lisa R.         Lisat@for.example.com

     Leslie T.       Starlt@example.com

     Mr. & Mrs. R.   homestead@example.org

     James T.        james@business.example

     Barbara S.      barbaraone@example.com

     Tina S.         Tsims@example.com

     Elizabeth P.    Lizjoe@for.example.net

     Bob K.          bob@example.org

     Pam M.          pmroads@example.net

        This is a sample of a Group E-mail List.
                  It is not a form.
```

Materials you will need

- The Seven Principles opposite, each written on its own folded index card. There should be enough cards so that each person can select one, even if some principles are repeated.
- A bowl

Time needed

- Fifteen minutes

Suggested Script for Leader

There are Seven Principles that seem to be at the core of every caregiver group's success. We've touched on several of them tonight, but they're important enough to spend a little time with. In this bowl are each of these principles on small folded cards. Some of them are in more than once, so that each of you can have one.

I'm going to pass around the bowl. Please select a folded card. Take a moment to read what is written on your card. This will be your principle.

Read each word. Be sure you understand the principle. See if you can think of an example of the principle at work.

When you are ready, read the card aloud to us as if you had made up that principle. [Group members read principles aloud.]

The principle you drew is the principle you will each be responsible for. This means making sure we all remember it in the course of our time together. We each need to keep that principle on our computer or our desk or our refrigerator and gently try to remind the rest of the group about it when we forget.

Note to Leader: Review the in-depth discussion of the Seven Principles on pages 33 to 35.

PRINCIPLE #1: Sharing Responsibility Is the Key to Not Burning Out.

PRINCIPLE #2: It Won't Work Unless Everyone Gains Something Personally.

PRINCIPLE #3: Know Your Limits and Stick to Them.

PRINCIPLE #4: There's No One Right Way to Do It.

PRINCIPLE #5: Anyone Who Wants to Help Should Be Encouraged.

PRINCIPLE #6: Trust the Group; Support Each Other.

PRINCIPLE #7: Keep Your Own Life in Good Working Order.

EXERCISE 11
Feelings, Part Two

Purpose
- To make it safe and easy for everyone to talk about their feelings
- To see how people are feeling now after the meeting
- To see how feelings can change

Materials you will need
- A bowl
- One index card (blank on both sides) for each person
- Pencils

Time needed

- Approximately fifteen minutes

Note to Leader: The feelings in the room have probably changed a great deal since the start of the meeting. People will probably be feeling more positive and not as alone. The person who is ill will probably be feeling more secure and not as guilty. Repeating this exercise can be a very positive way to end your meeting.

Again, do not call on people to read. Let them read their card when they feel ready. Make sure people do not rush this exercise. Should some of the feelings seem to be the same as earlier, do not stop the group to explore these feelings. They are a part of where your group is now.

If the person who is ill is still at the meeting, make sure he or she participates in this exercise.

Suggested Script for Leader

Please take a card. Be sure not to put your name on it.

Please print this sentence and then complete it: "What I am feeling now is   ."

Take your time. When you are finished, fold your card so the writing doesn't show and place your card in the bowl.

Note to Leader: Make sure everyone puts their card into the bowl and that each card is folded so the writing cannot be seen. Mix up the cards. Pass the bowl around.

Suggested Script for Leader

Please select a folded card.

This is now your card. Take a moment to read what is written on your card.

Make believe that you have written what is on your card. Take a minute and feel what the words say. If it is, in fact, your card, don't tell us.

When you are ready, read the card you selected to us as if it were your own.

If you have received a blank card, make up the sentence.

Closing

Suggested Script for Coordinator

If there are any questions about any of the forms or systems, I'll be happy to stay and answer them or help you work out who will be co-captains.

Suggested Script for Leader

[To the person who is ill:] *Well,* [your friend], *you now have a Share The Care group. Thank you for letting us be here for you and for each other.*

[To the group:] *Does anyone have anything they need to say or want to add?*

Thank you all for coming. It was wonderful to meet everyone and I look forward to getting to know all of you better.

Note to Leader and Coordinator: Congratulations! You did it! You have held your first and most difficult meeting. You have begun a process that will help you take care of your friend who is ill and take care of each other at the same time.

Tonight you have put into motion a new kind of family. It is a family that will keep its strength in the face of crisis, keep its health in the face of the tremendous job needed, and keep its humor while caring for someone seriously ill.

Some Final Tips for Leaders: What to do (say) if you're the leader and . . .

. . . someone wants to run the meeting his or her way:

"I'm sure a lot of really good ideas will emerge as we work together, but tonight is about a system that seems to have worked for a great number of groups, so tonight we're going to talk about the Share The Care system."

. . . someone brings up some huge issue that looks as if it will destroy the feelings and closeness that have been established:

Acknowledge what the person has to say but say, "Let's talk about it at another time."

. . . the real family is hurt or insulted:

Realize that this meeting may be the first time they have dealt with the seriousness of their loved one's condition and needs. Stress how lucky the sick person is to have such a supportive family and now such a support system of friends.

. . . people come into the meeting late:

If you've just started, you can stop and repeat. But if you're well into the introductions or beyond, you can't go back. The coordinator can make sure they have a name tag and the leader can briefly welcome them and say they'll catch up during the break.

. . . not enough people commit to being in the group:

Start with the people you have. Ask friends of friends, explore other possible people, have another meeting.

CHAPTER NINE

The Workbook: All the Materials You Need to Make Your Group Run

On the following pages, you will find all the forms (referred to in chapters 5 through 8) you need to create your own group. All of them are available to download, edit, and print out from the book Web site, http://www .sharethecare.org, or you can photocopy them from the book. (The enlargement percentage to use when photocopying blank forms onto standard-size 8½-by-11-inch paper is 150%.) With each form you will also find this information:

- An easy explanation of *what* it is, *why* you need it, and *how* it works
- Suggestions on how to complete it and who should do so
- A place to fill in the date on all forms, so you can easily tell if you have the most up-to-date version (it is vital to keep current)
- Easy-to-follow procedures for members to use, printed on the forms
- Tips for color-coding each form so it can be located easily

You will also find a checklist for the coordinator to help prepare the materials to be sent to the group following the first meeting. Remember, if you have more than fifteen people it would be wise to enlist the help of an assistant coordinator. Otherwise the amount of paperwork could take up a large portion of your time.

How to Use the Individual Data Form

What Is It?

The Individual Data Form starts on the next page and continues for the following two pages. It's a direct, simple way to collect a lot of information at your very first meeting. Please note, there is a blank version of Limits, Strengths, and Weaknesses (page 2) available on the Web site if you want to tailor your own version of skills or jobs that will be needed. It can be downloaded, edited, and printed out from http://www.sharethecare.org.

Why Do You Need It?

The information you collect in these pages serves to get everyone's vital statistics and assist in finding out who's good at what job. It is also used to create other important information forms you will need.

How Does It Work?

- Before the meeting, download and print these three pages. Photocopy a set for each person attending the meeting (on blue-tinted paper so they can easily be located) and staple them together. Have them ready to pass out for exercise 5 in the meeting. (Make a few extras to have on hand.)
- At the end of the meeting the completed forms will be collected by the coordinator. The information in them will be used to create the Telephone Tree, Yellow Pages, a Rotating Captain's Schedule, and the Group E-mail List.
- The information is the guide to matching up the right person for the right job. The coordinator can make photocopies of each set to give to members to use while they serve as captain. Or the coordinator (or assistant) can create a database of the information that is collected or create a chart that includes all of the information. This would work well if most people in the group have e-mail and are computer literate. The coordinator will have to determine what will work best for the group.

Note to <u>COORDINATOR</u>:
• Use in first meeting.
• Copy on blue-tinted paper.
• Staple together with pages 2, 3.

Date: _____

S H A R E   T H E   C A R E

INDIVIDUAL DATA FORM

(page 1)

Name _____

Address: Street _____ Apt. _____

City _____ State _____ Zip _____

Home phone: (   ) _____

Work phone: (   ) _____

Service phone: (   ) _____

Other phone: (weekend home) (   ) _____

Fax: (   ) _____

Cell: (   ) _____

E-mail: _____

Occupation: _____

Do you have a car?   yes (   )   no (   ) If not, can you drive?   yes (   )   no (   )

Can you participate as a Share The Care member?   yes (   )   no (   )

If you feel you cannot participate as a Share The Care member,
can you commit to being a free-floater?   yes (   )   no (   )

AVAILABILITY: Are there any days or specific hours when you know you would <u>NOT BE</u>
<u>AVAILABLE?</u> Please indicate in the chart below:

Time	Monday	Tuesday	Wednesday	Thursday	Friday	Saturday	Sunday
9:00 A.M. 1:00 P.M.							
1:00 P.M. 5:00 P.M.							
5:00 P.M. 10:00 P.M.							
10:00 P.M. Overnight							

OTHER: (Specific dates)

<table>
<tr><td colspan="2">
NOTE TO <u>COORDINATOR</u>:
• Use in first meeting.
• Copy on blue-tinted paper.
• Staple together with pages 1, 3.
</td></tr>
</table>

Date: _____

INDIVIDUAL DATA FORM
YOUR LIMITS, STRENGTHS, AND WEAKNESSES   (page 2)

Name _____

This form is designed to try to find the right person for the job whenever possible.

Where do you fit in when it comes to the following areas?

Remember, it's okay not to like something or not to be good at another thing. Someone else in the group may like to do what you don't. Rate yourself on the following:

IN DEALING WITH	I'M TERRIFIC	I'M GOOD	I'M FAIR	DON'T CALL ON ME
Emergencies				
Paperwork Organization				
Insurance Forms				
Hospitals				
Talking to Doctors				
Physical Tasks				
Cooking Special Foods				
Research				
Xeroxing Paperwork				
Listening and Taking Notes				
Asking Questions				
Needles				
Blood				
Making Appointments				
Shopping (Grocery)				
Shopping (Personal Items)				
Hiring Help				
Firing Help				
Housecleaning				
Finding Solutions to Problems				

NOTE TO <u>COORDINATOR</u>:
• Use in first meeting.
• Copy on blue-tinted paper.
• Staple together with pages 1, 2.

Date: _____

INDIVIDUAL DATA FORM
YOUR LIMITS, STRENGTHS, AND WEAKNESSES

(page 3)

Name _____

In your own words, is there anything else that you want to tell us about
what you like to do, are a "star" at doing, don't want to do, or abhor?

I am truly great at:

I absolutely cannot deal with:

Special skills and hobbies:

Tip for Coordinator: Photocopy all copies of filled-in Individual Data Forms (3 pages) or your own tailor-made Individual Data Form on blue-tinted paper so they can easily be distinguished from other materials.

How to Create the Rotating Captain's Schedule

What Is It?

The six-month Rotating Captain's Schedule tells all members the specific weeks that they will serve as a captain. Two co-captains are assigned to work together for each week. *Very important:* A caregiver group week is Monday, Tuesday, Wednesday, Thursday, Friday, Saturday, *through and including* Sunday.

Why Do You Need It?

The captains are vital to running the group, which cannot function without them. The captains are in charge of scheduling *everything* during their assigned week. This includes handling any emergency that might arise for the person who is ill during their assigned week. *Being captain is the most important job you will have as a member.*

How Does It Work?

- At the first meeting, a member can sign up to serve with someone, or the coordinator will assign teams of co-captains.
- Each team will serve a week at a time on a rotating basis for a six-month period.
- The coordinator is responsible for updating the Rotating Captain's Schedule and sending it out to all members one month before the old one expires.
- *The rule is this:* If a captain absolutely cannot fill his or her week, he or she must (1) notify the co-captain, (2) find a replacement, (3) let the group know via e-mail or Telephone Tree.

NOTE TO <u>COORDINATOR</u>:
This schedule can be filled in, saved, and edited online, then printed.
• Copy on pink-tinted paper.

Date: _____

SHARE THE CARE

ROTATING CAPTAIN'S SCHEDULE

A Share The Care week is: Monday, Tuesday, Wednesday, Thursday, Friday, Saturday, through and including Sunday.

IMPORTANT: If you absolutely cannot be captain for a specific week you must
1. Notify your co-captain,
2. Find a replacement, *and*
3. Let the group know via e-mail or the Telephone Tree.

CAPTAINS	DATES (FOR WEEKS OF:)
1. 2.	
1. 2.	
1. 2.	
1. 2.	
1. 2.	
1. 2.	
1. 2.	

> **Tip for Coordinator:** Photocopy the completed schedule on pink-tinted paper so it can be easily located. Mark your calendar to remind yourself when to update it. See also the helpful tips and charts at the end of the chapter (pages 124–37).

How to Create Your Own Caring Schedule

What Is It?

The Caring Schedule is a weekly schedule used by the captains. It's an easy plan for scheduling everything that will be needed by the person who is ill.

Why Do You Need It?

As a captain you will use it to fit members into specific needed time slots. You will also need to give a copy of the completed schedule to the person who is ill so he or she will know whom to expect and when to expect them, and to relieve any anxieties he or she might have about the upcoming week.

How Does It Work?

- The scheduling process begins on the *Thursday prior to the Monday* of the week being planned, when one of the Captains calls the person who is ill to find out what is needed for the upcoming week.
- By Saturday the schedule must be completed and ready to begin on Monday.
- After you speak to the person who is ill, make a priority list of what will be needed *before* you start calling the group members. *Get the most important jobs filled first.* For example, use this order of importance:

1. Hospital admissions
2. Doctor, therapy appointments (make sure you get specific times)
3. Prescriptions to be filled
4. Making meals
5. Sleepovers
6. Help with bath or shower
7. Errands, shopping
8. Repairs
9. Paperwork, insurance forms
10. Entertainment

NOTE TO COORDINATOR:
Copy on pink-tinted paper.

Hospital: _____
Address: _____

Room: _____ Tel: _____
Visiting Hrs: _____

Date: _____
Captain: _____
Captain: _____

SHARE THE CARE
CARING SCHEDULE

DATES							
TIME	MONDAY	TUESDAY	WEDNESDAY	THURSDAY	FRIDAY	SATURDAY	SUNDAY
9:00 A.M. 1:00 P.M.							
1:00 P.M. 5:00 P.M.							
5:00 P.M. 10:00 P.M.							
Overnight							

- If you cannot get all jobs filled by members, call on free-floaters and/or real family.
- *Important note to captains:* During your week, carry a copy of your schedule, the Yellow Pages, and the Telephone Tree, in case anything unexpected should arise and/or additional help is needed.

Tip for Coordinator: Make blank photocopies of this form on pink-tinted paper for easy location. All members should have five to ten blank copies for use when they are captains.

How to Create Your Own Telephone Tree

What Is It?

In case of an emergency, the Telephone Tree is the most efficient way to reach everyone in the group without having to make more than two telephone calls each.

It contains *all telephone numbers* (including area codes) where members can be reached at any time: home, work, cell phone, weekend home, fax number, and any other number.

Why Do You Need It?

You never know when you may need to contact all the members of the group, and sending out an e-mail may not get the quick response needed. Examples of information you will be able to pass along quickly using the Telephone Tree:

- The person who is ill was just taken to the emergency room.
- The person who is ill does not want to be disturbed by phone calls.
- The group needs to call a meeting right away.

How Does It Work?

- Put the name of the person who is ill at the top of the tree
- Put the name of the person with the most daily contact in Position A. This person might be your friend's roommate, spouse, or best friend.

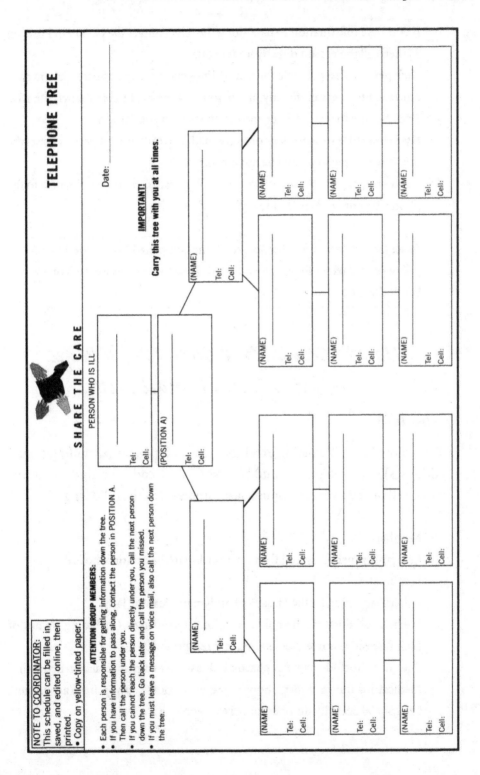

TELEPHONE TREE

Date: _____

IMPORTANT!
Carry this tree with you at all times.

SHARE THE CARE

NOTE TO COORDINATOR:
This schedule can be filled in, saved, and edited online, then printed.
• Copy on yellow-tinted paper.

ATTENTION GROUP MEMBERS:

• Each person is responsible for getting information down the tree.
• If you have information to pass along, contact the person in POSITION A. Then call the person under you.
• If you cannot reach the person directly under you, call the next person down the tree. Go back later and call the person you missed.
• If you must leave a message on voice mail, also call the next person down the tree.

PERSON WHO IS ILL

Tel:
Cell:

(POSITION A)

Tel:
Cell:

(NAME)

Tel:
Cell:

(NAME)

Tel:
Cell:

(NAME)

Tel:
Cell:

(NAME)

Tel:
Cell:

(NAME)

Tel:
Cell:

(NAME)

Tel:
Cell:

(NAME)

Tel:
Cell:

(NAME)

Tel:
Cell:

(NAME)

Tel:
Cell:

(NAME)

Tel:
Cell:

(NAME)

Tel:
Cell:

(NAME)

Tel:
Cell:

- If you have information to pass along the tree, contact the person in Position A, then call the person directly under you.
- Each person is responsible for getting information down the tree. If you cannot reach the person directly under you, call the next person down the tree. Then be sure to go back later and call the person you missed.
- If you have to leave a message on voice mail, also call the next person down the tree (the first person could be out of town).
- Carry your copy of this tree with you at all times. Keep extra copies next to the phone in your weekend home, office, and car.

Tip for Coordinator: Make photocopies of the completed Telephone Tree on yellow-tinted paper for easy location. Make several copies for each member of the group.

How to Create Your Own Yellow Pages and the Group E-mail List

What Is It?

The Yellow Pages is a listing of all the names, addresses (including e-mail addresses), and telephone numbers with area codes (including home, work, cell phone, weekend house, fax numbers) for the following:

- Members
- Real family members, and their relationship to the person who is ill
- Free-floaters
- Other: babysitter, landlord, super, handyman, cleaning lady
- Medical: all doctors, therapists, surgeons, technicians (including names of their respective nurses, secretaries, and receptionists)
- Pharmacy: include name of pharmacist (as well as any special instructions)
- Medical insurance information: name of advocate, group insurance numbers, Social Security number for person who is ill

NOTE TO <u>COORDINATOR</u>:
This form can be filled in, saved, and edited online, then printed.
• Copy on yellow-tinted paper.
• Staple together pages 1–5.

S H A R E   T H E   C A R E

YELLOW PAGES

Date: _____

CAREGIVER GROUP MEMBERS	(INCLUDE AREA CODE)		
NAME & ADDRESS	TELEPHONE	CELL NUMBER	E-MAIL

P. 2 — Copy on yellow-tinted paper.			Date: _____
REAL FAMILY		(INCLUDE AREA CODE)	
NAME, RELATIONSHIP, & ADDRESS	**TELEPHONE**	**CELL NUMBER**	**E-MAIL**

P. 3 — Copy on yellow-tinted paper.   Date: _____

FREE-FLOATERS   (INCLUDE AREA CODE)

NAME & ADDRESS	TELEPHONE	CELL NUMBER	E-MAIL

OTHER (SUPERINTENDENT, BABYSITTER, HANDYMAN, LANDLORD)

NAME & ADDRESS	TELEPHONE	CELL NUMBER	E-MAIL

P. 4 — Copy on yellow-tinted paper.   Date: _____

MEDICAL (INCLUDE NAME OF NURSE, RECEPTIONIST, SECRETARY)   (INCLUDE AREA CODE)

DOCTOR'S NAME & ADDRESS (include specialty)	E-MAIL	TELEPHONE

P. 5 — Copy on yellow-tinted paper		Date: _____
PHARMACY (INCLUDE NAME OF PHARMACIST)		(INCLUDE AREA CODE)
NAME & ADDRESS	**TELEPHONE**	**FAX AND E-MAIL**
MEDICAL INSURANCE		(INCLUDE AREA CODE)
NAME & ADDRESS	**TELEPHONE**	**FAX AND E-MAIL**

*Be sure to include
Name of insurance
Group insurance number
Social Security number
Any other specific company identification

Why Do You Need It?

Your group's Yellow Pages will contain all the names and numbers of anyone you might need in order to help the person who is ill *at any time of the day or night*. The group e-mail list will allow members to communicate non-emergency messages to everyone in the group at once.

How Does It Work?

- Members carry these Yellow Pages with them (along with a copy of the Telephone Tree) at all times. (If you have a weekend home, an office, or a car, it is also a good idea to leave an extra copy there.)
- A copy of the Yellow Pages is also kept in a designated place (by each telephone) at the home of the person who is ill.
- Have everyone enter all the members' e-mail addresses in their computer address books as a group.

Tip for Coordinator: You will need to schedule some time with the person who is ill in order to collect some of this information from his or her address book, e-mail address book, Palm Pilot, Rolodex, or papers. Photocopy the completed Yellow Pages on yellow-tinted paper for easy location. Make several copies for each member of the group and the patient. If members do not have e-mail, make sure they are contacted by phone. This can be done by the person sending the message or by a prearranged volunteer.

After the Meeting

Checklist for the Coordinator: Using the information you collect in the first meeting from the Individual Data Forms, you will put together the following materials and send them to each member of the group (including the person who is ill). Each packet should contain:

- A cover letter. You may use the one on page 120 as a model or photocopy it as a form letter and fill in the blanks.

- A guide to the Share The Care forms and a copy of the Seven Principles. (We suggest you photocopy pages 121–23.) Be sure to fill in the name of the person who is ill, in the blanks on all three pages.
- A completed Rotating Captain's Schedule for a six-month period photocopied on *pink-tinted paper*. Remember, *you* are responsible for updating this schedule *one month* before it expires. *Mark your calendar.*
- A completed Telephone Tree photocopied on *yellow-tinted paper*. Send three or four copies to each member (check the tree to see how many phones each one has and send at least one copy for each phone listed).
- A completed Yellow Pages photocopied on *yellow-tinted paper*. Send several sets of these pages to each member (check to see how many phones each one has). *Be sure to have a set near the phone and another near the computer of the person who is ill.*
- Print or photocopy the Group E-mail List on *yellow-tinted paper* to include with (but not attached to) the Yellow Pages.
- Five to ten *blank* copies of the Caring Schedule photocopied on *pink-tinted paper,* to be used by each member when captain. Keep a supply of these on hand.
- A set of everyone's *filled-in* Individual Data Forms photocopied on *blue-tinted paper* (all three pages for each member). To be used by members when captain, these forms will help them find the right person for the job. Or, if you prefer, create a chart that breaks out the basic information for quick reference.

Date:

Dear Group Member,

It's great to have you as a member of _____'s Share The Care Family.

This package contains all the forms and information you will need to help get the group off to a great beginning and keep it running efficiently.

I suggest you keep everyone's Individual Data Form information in a folder where it can be easily located. Because this is *private information,* please make sure you keep it in a secure place and do not share it with anyone outside the group. Keep the Telephone Tree and Yellow Pages with you at all times so you can reach other group members, family members, or medical personnel involved with _____'s care. Also, it's a good idea to keep a set of copies at your weekend home, your office, and in your car.

I have color-coded the forms and enclosed a brief explanation to refresh your memory. Also included are the Seven Principles that we discussed at the meeting. Please try to keep these important points in mind as our work begins.

If you have any questions, please call and I'll do my best to help.

Warm regards,

Coordinator's name:

Telephone:

E-mail:

A Guide to the Enclosed Forms

Individual Data Forms (Blue)

These are copies of everyone's three-page form for your use when you serve as a captain. The information in them will be helpful in locating the best person for a particular job.

They are especially useful when there are a lot of us in the group who don't know each other very well (or not at all). Later, as we get to know each other better, we probably won't need to rely on these forms so much and will instinctively know whom to call first. This is *private information,* so please keep it in a secure place.

Rotating Captain's Schedule (Pink)

This schedule lists the weeks you are to serve as a captain and who your co-captain will be. It might be a good idea to mark your calendars now and to give your co-captain a call and get to know her or him better, especially if you only just met at the meeting.

There are three important points for you to remember if you absolutely cannot be a co-captain the week you are assigned: (1) you must find a replacement among the other members to switch with you for that week; (2) you must notify your co-captain of the change and who your replacement will be; and (3) you must let the group know via e-mail or telephone.

The coordinator will be sending everyone another Rotating Captain's Schedule one month before this one is due to expire.

Caring Schedule (Pink)

These blank forms are for you to use when you are captain in order to schedule everything   needs during your week!

A suggested way to use this schedule:

1. One of the captains calls   to find out what will be needed for the upcoming week (i.e., doctors, therapy appointments, treatments, hospital ad-

missions, shopping, errands). This process should begin on the *Thursday prior to the Monday* of the week being planned.

2. Your schedule, ideally, should be completed by Saturday and ready to begin on Monday.

3. After speaking to   , make a priority list of what will be needed *before* you and the co-captain start calling other members. Get the most important jobs filled first. For example, these items are in priority order:

   • Hospital admissions
   • Doctor or therapy appointments (make sure you get specific times)
   • Prescriptions to be filled
   • Making meals
   • Sleepovers
   • Help with bath or shower
   • Errands, shopping, housekeeping
   • Repairs
   • Paperwork, insurance forms
   • Entertainment

4. If you cannot get all jobs filled by members, then call on free-floaters and/or real family.

5. Remember to give a copy of the completed schedule to   so he or she will know whom to expect and when to expect them. This will also help relieve any anxieties he or she might have about the upcoming week.

6. While you are captain, carry a copy of your schedule with you everywhere in the event anything unexpected should arise and/or additional help is needed.

Telephone Tree (Yellow)

Using this tree system, we can pass along information or news quickly to everyone in the group without having to make more than two phone calls each.

Some points to remember:

1. Each person is responsible for getting information down the tree.
2. If you cannot reach the person(s) directly under you, call the next per-

son down the tree. Then be sure to go back later and call the person you missed.

3. If you have to leave a message on voice mail, also call the next person down the tree (the first person could be out of town).

4. If you have information to pass along the tree, contact the person in Position A, then call the person(s) directly under you.

5. Carry the tree with you at all times and keep copies in your weekend home, your office, and your car.

Yellow Pages (Yellow)

This directory contains the names and numbers of anyone you might need to contact in order to help   at any time of the day or night. Carry it with you at all times and keep copies at other locations where you spend time.

Group E-mail List (Yellow)

Attached for your convenience is a list of everyone's e-mail addresses. Please enter them into your computer *as a group* so you can easily e-mail the entire group at once. Also, please note those members who have no e-mail and the person assigned to inform them of important e-mail notices. This is in case you know the contact person is unavailable; then you can call those without e-mail yourself.

The Seven Principles

PRINCIPLE #1:	Sharing Responsibility Is the Key to Not Burning Out.
PRINCIPLE #2:	It Won't Work Unless Everyone Gains Something Personally.
PRINCIPLE #3:	Know Your Limits and Stick to Them.
PRINCIPLE #4:	There's No One Right Way to Do It.
PRINCIPLE #5:	Anyone Who Wants to Help Should Be Encouraged.
PRINCIPLE #6:	Trust the Group; Support Each Other.
PRINCIPLE #7:	Keep Your Own Life in Good Working Order.

Note to Coordinator: Some of the following information should be shared with the group once you have things running smoothly (Task Chart Sample, Captain Tips). These ideas will make more sense to the group members once they have started the process of sharing the care. Several of the other ideas are for use later on as you need them (Specialist Captains, Problem-Solving Chart). The Internet information may need to go only to the person setting up the communications system.

Useful Charts and Tips to Share

Useful Charts

Many skills we learn in the workplace can easily be translated into making things run more smoothly in your Share The Care group. Be open to suggestions from members who may have an interesting new way of resolving issues, charting jobs, or keeping records. We want to share with you some that have proved very helpful in a number of circumstances.

TASK CHART SAMPLE

In the beginning, when captains and the person who is ill are figuring out exactly what jobs need to be handled, it might be helpful to write out the jobs for following weeks' captains. These will most likely be ongoing tasks. This will save time and effort, and it will create continuity so the person who is ill doesn't have to go through the process again and again as captains rotate. Jeanie's Share The Care group devised a chart of her needs that made it simpler for the captains to make their calls. They had a clear and specific breakdown so they could explain jobs to the members more easily and then just fill in the names. See the sample on page 125.

PROBLEM-SOLVING CHART

Sometimes when things get complicated and confusing, it helps to sort out our thoughts on paper. Cappy's group devised a Problem-Solving Chart that can easily be created on your computer. You can break it out in this

THINGS JEANIE NEEDS		
WHAT TASK	**WHAT IS INVOLVED**	**WHO**
Transportation	• space in your vehicle for walker or wheel chair • assist with getting from house to car and then to appointment (1st thing in the morning appt means helping to get ready to leave the house)	
Cleaning	• this is more spot cleaning, dishes, putting things away • laundry	
Meal preparation	• be there at lunchtime to help fix a lunch • be around to assist with lunch • once in a while do a dinner for relief for the family	
Being present	• maybe just sitting (this is to have someone in the house) • reading to Jeanie • renting movies	
Help with personal care	• bathing, dressing, personal care	
Making phone calls	• calling various docs to make appointments, get equipment • following up with needed calls	
Shopping	• being there when groceries arrive • purchasing necessary items • taking Jeanie shopping • putting away groceries	
Yard work	• seasonal jobs, raking, weeding, pruning . . .	
Recording/ storytelling	• recording anecdotes • asking questions • getting information	
Other	• massage • painting • fun outings	

way: Category, Item, Issue, and Action By. Then you can fill it in and e-mail it to the group to discuss and implement. Try this next time when things get overwhelming. There's a sample on pages 127–28.

Captain Tips

A group in California bears the unusual name Share The Care Sangha. *Sangha* is one of the three jewels in the Buddhist tradition; the word refers to the community of people who practice together. The spiritual practice in this case is that of love, compassion, awareness, and service. They care for a man named Andy, who has neuroendocrine cancer, and the circle supports his wife and children. They have ten core members with fifty free-floaters (including two teens). Their coordinator, Ann, oversees and manages the captains. The following suggestions have come from their first eight weeks of captaining. See if any would be helpful for your group to adopt, or perhaps they will spark your imagination to create your own version.

Share The Care Sangha Captain Tips

- Some pairs of captains have found it helpful to divide their work and have one make the initial calls to fill the week's needs while the other one acts as the contact during the week for spontaneous needs.

- As you find out information about a free-floater that might be helpful to future captains when calling (for example, availability info, job preferences), please forward it to the coordinator to include it in the reports for the next week's captains.

- It is helpful if household members explain the week's needs directly to the person who is going to make most of the calls. That way they can give suggestions about whom to call for which jobs.

- It is important to keep any of our captains' stress away from the family. If there are frustrations, call the other captain or coordinator.

- It is *very* important to emphasize timeliness to the members. Time is essential in order for his wife to get Andy to an appointment.

- Because Andy's immune system is not strong, members who are not feel-

PROBLEM-SOLVING CHART
Date:

CATEGORY	ITEM	ISSUE	ACTION BY:
Fire Island	Closing	Cappy is planning to go out to Fire Island late next week with Eileen and Sheila, et al, I believe. It's my understanding that Jim is going to join them toward the end of the stay and they will close the house at the end of the trip.	Jim Sheila Eileen Possibly others . . .
Primary care physician	Dr. S. Jones	Roger set up an appointment for Cappy with Dr. Jones. I believe the proper forms have been filed with the insurance so that he's listed as Cappy's primary care physician. All treatments should be referred to his office—he will make appropriate referrals and Cappy's bills will be covered by insurance.	Roger Pat
Chest congestion	Dr. S. Jones	Cappy has some problem developing in her lungs. An X-ray was taken and Dr. Jones has prescribed an antibiotic course; Dom has advised us to watch this carefully as Cappy's condition can mask symptoms of a more serious infection. Christina is aware of this and we're watching it.	Everyone
MRI	New MRI	It's vitally important that we get an updated MRI. Status is as follows: 1. We have in hand her 3/21 post-surgical MRI. 2. We have in hand her 4/14 MRI when she was admitted to ER. 3. We have a request into Dr. Black's office for the 5/24 MRI that that was done when she re-entered the treatment in Houston. We have been promised a set by early next week. 4. I will be seeing Cappy on Saturday and will arrange to schedule an MRI appointment for next week. Sheila will accompany Cappy . . . otherwise we will need a volunteer.	Steve Sheila Possible another volunteer
Speech therapy	Payment	Anne arranged speech therapy for Cappy. She's been going three times a week. We now need to determine how Cappy's getting reimbursed from insurance. Anne was looking into this issue. We need to know whether help is needed from Pat. Anne: please advise.	Anne

PROBLEM-SOLVING CHART

(page 2)

CATEGORY	ITEM	ISSUE	ACTION BY:
Physical therapy	Arrange physical therapy	Regardless of the snafu of insurance authorization, there's no question Cappy would benefit from PT. Jean is PT Captain—please go ahead and schedule a preliminary appointment for Cappy. SUGGESTION: While there might be someone who would come to Cappy's apartment, going out to an appointment is an important and helpful part of her day. Jean—please see if you can arrange an appointment with a therapist who's within reasonable rolling distance of Cappy's apartment so she can go over there for PT.	Jean
Cappy diet	Healthful & healing diet	Dom and the nutritionist in Colorado suggested a healthful, supportive diet for treatment of a brain tumor. There is a two-step process here: 1. Eileen, Dom, Sheila, & Steve (and possibly others) need to sit down with Cappy and discuss the diet issue. We need to get her to understand the necessity and importance of this dietary regimen and enroll her in the program. 2. Once she's enrolled, we need to put a program in place so she follows the diet. Eileen and Ric have volunteered to co-captain her diet and Patsy was hired specifically to help with the cooking.	Eileen Ric Patsy & Everyone
Biofeedback	Jim R.	Cappy has been having weekly Thursday sessions with a biofeedback practitioner. She has expressed a positive reaction to these treatments and would like them to continue past the "four weeks" Jim originally suggested. Would this week's captain speak to Jim and make sure he can continue to see her in the coming weeks?	This week's captain(s)
Healing	Richard	Richard comes in every Wednesday for a two-hour session with Cappy. He's now developed quite a following and books pretty much the whole day with other members of the Brain Trust. Cappy would like these sessions to continue.	Everyone who sees Richard

ing well or who may have anything contagious should get a replacement if possible (call the captain). They can call Andy's wife or the coordinator first if they are not sure.

- A reminder of dietary requests if you are bringing/making food: Fish, seafood, or vegetarian. Non-wheat, non-dairy, and low-sugar. (Alter to fit other patients' needs.)

- When calling a member, if you have to leave a message, tell them to feel free to return the call, or you will call them back later if they prefer. Some captains found that making a second call was more successful than just waiting for a callback.

- If a helper does call back and the job was already filled, go ahead and fill that helper in for the following week, or pass on a note to the next captain that they are willing to help.

- Many Sangha members didn't specify everything they are willing to help with, or didn't even fill out the full form. In other words, even if they only checked "meals," they may be willing to do other things, such as give rides, be a home-helper, or some other specific need. It doesn't hurt to ask.

- Once the needs for the week are filled, please get a list of the "jobs" and the members filling them to the patient's wife, a copy to the captains for the next week, and a copy to the coordinator (via phone or e-mail).

- If captains or coordinator wish to use the Yahoo group for requesting help, please run the e-mail by Andy's wife first, if possible, for the sake of privacy. The Yahoo group is composed of dozens of additional friends and family who are not part of the Sangha.

Specialist Captains

At one point Cappy's Brain Trust captains were nearly burnt out by her fast-paced illness and emergencies. The group started using "Specialist Captains" to make sure the many facets of her life didn't fall through the cracks. Once the specialists were in place the group continued with regular weekly rotating captains, but their jobs became manageable again. If your group is having difficulties it might be a good idea to break down specific jobs into permanent assignments, especially such crucial issues as finances, medical insurance, and medical contacts. Here's how they did it:

FINANCIAL: This captain handled all finances, collected Cappy's mail, sorted and paid her bills, and balanced her checkbook.

LEGAL: A member who was an attorney made sure all of her directives, will, and other papers were in order. He also had her power of attorney.

MEDICAL CLAIM INSURANCE: The member who handled this job lived in New Jersey. You don't have to live close by to handle this very important job.

SUMMERHOUSE RENTAL: Two people very familiar with the property made all the arrangements so the rental commitment could be honored.

SPEECH THERAPY: One member found an approved therapist and scheduled members to take Cappy to appointments as well as help her to practice exercises.

PHYSICAL THERAPY: Same as above.

MEDICAL: Chiefly handled by three members of the core group. Calling doctors and going to medical appointments, they were also the medical proxies.

COOKING/DIET: Two members agreed to oversee information, shopping, and preparation of healthy meals as advised by the nutritionist.

RAMPS: One member researched and purchased a collapsible metal ramp to get her up and down lobby stairs after we obtained approvals from the building's board. Another member built a wooden ramp to provide access to the terrace garden from the apartment.

TERRACE GARDEN: The member who created the magnificent garden took it on as a permanent assignment. He visited daily to water, clip, and tend to the flowers as well as help with whatever else might be needed.

COMMUNICATIONS: As doctors changed or new ones were added, our Yellow Pages were in need of serious updates, so two members handled this project. The revised version included new information about which emergency room we should visit if needed.

AMBULETTE SERVICES/VISITS:	One person took charge of all ambulette arrangements to get her to doctors' appointments or visits with her dad.
RELIEF AIDES:	Three members collaborated to screen and hire applicants for this position.
BUSINESS COMMITMENTS:	Two members covered all her ongoing creative business throughout the year.

Technology: Ideas for Broader Communication

But Don't Give Up Connecting in Person and by Phone

Back in the late 1980s and early 1990s, when we were helping Susan, e-mail was not even a dream, much less an option, for the Funny Family. Today, electronic communication allows us to stay connected with everyone even if they're on the opposite coast or the other side of the world. Technology lets us document and keep important information up-to-date without a lot of hassle. Just don't let it be the *only* way you communicate. Cherish the connections you make with your fellow members by phone and in person. (You can't give someone, in tears after a traumatic time in the ER, a hug through an e-mail.) Overlooking the personal part of "being there" for another caregiver would be a terrible loss for you both. Please be sure to remind your group of this every so often.

Sorting Out Some Options for Your Group

There are many options for communication, and only you will be able to determine which will work best for your particular group. The best option will depend on the answers to questions such as these: Does everyone in the group have a computer? Does everyone have e-mail and Internet access? How large is the group? How widespread (geographically) is the group? Steve (from Cappy's Brain Trust) and Jennifer (from Share The Care Sangha) offer the following information and advice to help you make informed decisions about using e-mail and blogs, and about communicating ideas if your group is very large.

E-MAIL, BLOGS, AND WEB SITES, BY STEVE

Group E-mail

Steve recalls the journey of the Brain Trust through a long trail of group e-mails:

> I was sitting here this morning re-reading some of the Brain Trust e-mails chronologically from last year. We were all excellent communicators, and I found reading them really took me back into the experience in a very vivid way. Who each of us is came through in our individual notes. Our fears, our uncertainties, certainties, opinions, hopes, beliefs, concerns—it's all there. I just felt like writing you a note to mention that in reading the e-mails I think everyone in Cappy's life was absolutely HEROIC in their efforts. Over the past few months I'd forgotten all the emergencies and setbacks and the way the group responded to everything we were dealt. There's no question in my mind that she got the best possible support and help any human being could ask for.

Web mail can generally be set up with various distribution groups. So after initially entering every member's e-mail address, you can assign individuals to certain categories, which can be used as separate e-mail lists. Once this has been set up, you simply click on the name you've assigned to the e-mail group and your message will go out to all individuals in that group. For example, with Cappy's Brain Trust, there were two different groups: a "general" group list for information, updates, and schedules, and a "core" group made up of a half-dozen members who were handling her personal finances, had medical proxies, and were involved in key decisions.

For most groups, e-mail updates will become the main avenue for keeping friends and relatives abreast of the group's progress and needs. Regular updates and requests for assistance can be made (generally by a family member, the coordinator, the captains), and e-mailed to everyone. Here are a few tips:

- It is important to maintain accurate e-mail addresses for everyone. Assign one or two people (perhaps the ones responsible for updating the Yellow Pages) to the task of keeping the list current.

- As a matter of courtesy, it's good to put your group's e-mail addresses on the "Bcc" (blind copy) line instead of the "To" section. This prevents everyone's e-mail address from being revealed all over the place when the letter is forwarded.

- Many e-mail programs and Web hosts will not allow e-mail messages to be sent out to large groups of people at once. A typical limit is 99. Share The Care Sangha tried to use Yahoo Mail and were unable to send even 50 at a time. (For more on the Yahoo Mail, see the communications ideas from Jennifer later in this chapter).

Groups will discover that there are good and bad things about e-mail. The good thing? It makes it easy to stay in touch and will give you a lasting record of everything that happened. The bad thing? It can easily get out of control. If everyone feels compelled to reply to every e-mail that's sent, the volume of mail can easily get up into the thousands. With e-mail it gets easy to lose the personal connection. Huge volumes of e-mail are no substitute for "face time."

Blogs

One way to avoid overwhelming the inbox is to set up a Web log (called a "blog"). These days, almost all Internet Service Providers offer some kind of free or low-cost blog option, and there are a large number of service options.

1. *Public blogs.* These are the most common type of blog. They allow anyone who finds or knows the URL (the address) to log onto your blog and read the contents. If you want to share your group's story with other people, you might want to do this. Sometimes a well-meaning soul who comes across your address might offer some advice or information that could be invaluable. On the other hand, if you're planning to post medicine schedules and private information, you may not want a public blog.

2. *Private blogs.* As the name implies, private blogs block people who don't know the address and password from logging onto the site.

3. *Single host/multiple host.* Who has permission to enter information? Most blog sites offer users a limited choice of options—either "one user" or "open to the public." But some sites let you list everyone who can enter primary information.

4. *Feedback.* Like the Host option, you can set up a blog so anyone can respond or no one can respond. For a Share The Care group, letting everyone respond allows a powerful sharing forum that will keep your personal e-mail box from filling up. And the record of progress is there for everyone to see, so as new members join the group they can go back to early blog entries and get caught up with what's been happening.

As one of the hottest new Internet options, there are thousands of blog hosts. If you go to an Internet search engine (such as Google) and type "blog hosts," you'll get an extensive directory of hosting options.

Our advice? A blog hosting site is a big plus. Select one that isn't free. ("Free" blog hosts generally capture your address and then bombard you with spam. You'll rue the day you gave them your e-mail information.) For as little as $25 a year or as much as $10 a month, you'll find blog hosts that will give you a wide range of privacy, security, and e-mail options.

Even if some of your group members don't have an e-mail address, they can still connect with a blog. By using a friend's computer or a public-access computer, they can type the URL in the address line and stay in touch through the Internet.

FREE WEB SITE FOR PATIENTS

Jeanie's Share The Care group in Oregon has been using a free Web site to post information and pictures so her wide circle of friends, family, and group members can stay informed. There is a guest book on the site so visitors can leave short messages for her. The Web site is run by a nonprofit organization called CaringBridge. See http://www.CaringBridge.org for more information.

IDEAS FOR MANAGING COMMUNICATIONS
FOR A LARGE GROUP, BY JENNIFER

Both the Share The Care Sangha participants and all the other friends and family members who needed to be kept up-to-date felt the need for communication. This group turned out to be extremely large, and needed various levels of communication.

The initial invitation to join the group went out by e-mail to hundreds of people, both near and far. This general e-mail list was maintained on the family's computer (with their e-mail program), and regular updates went out to everyone. Since Web servers won't usually allow e-mails to be sent out to large lists of people, our list was broken down into several distribution lists of ninety addresses each. This system worked fairly well, but managing all of the undelivered (bounced) mail, address changes, and resends was time-consuming. One solution for this could be the use of free or inexpensive software, which allows one to send newsletters or bulletins to anyone who's requested to be added to the list. Often, the subscription process can be as simple as sending a "Reply" to the invitation e-mail. Such programs usually have a process for automatically handling undeliverable e-mails.

The second need for communication was among all those actively participating as group members. This too proved to be a large e-mail list, and efforts were made to get everyone onto Yahoo Groups so all had ways of contacting each other and staying in the loop. "However," Jennifer reports, "we were unable to use Yahoo Groups effectively since only about half of the members subscribed. Groups have great potential *if* everyone subscribes. While some e-mail was used, our captains mostly contacted members by phone. Though this worked, it took much more time, and the group didn't get the benefit of the full exchange of communications."

Using a Database
In order to give the captains the best information available on the interests and availabilities of the members, we created a database with Microsoft Access. One advantage of a database is that you can create very specific reports with the exact information needed. For example, from the same

database we could generate a simple phone list of all the members alpha-betized by first name, a report of contact and availability information con-solidated into a few pages, or lists of each type of job with names and degree of their interest in that job.

Another benefit of a database is that the information can be easily up-dated and reprinted when someone joins the group or changes their pref-erences. Not only are databases invaluable when trying to keep track of all the information in a large group, they also cut down on the time, expense, and amount of paper used in copying.

Microsoft Access is a somewhat difficult database for beginners to use—there are easier and less expensive programs available. (Ebase is one such free database application to consider.) A great resource for informa-tion on inexpensive software is http://www.techsoup.org, which focuses on technology for nonprofits. The type of software used by nonprofits fits nicely with the kind of information that needs to be tracked in a Share The Care group.

Using Yahoo Groups

There are many different types of community-building applications avail-able on the Internet. Yahoo Groups is one such service, and the one we used. It combines e-mail communications with Web site features. The main advantages of Yahoo Groups are as follows:

- List owners, and moderators chosen by the owner, have some control over the Web site options (chat, files, photos, links, database, polls, and calendar), and can choose to approve or deny messages and/or members.
- Individuals maintain their own profile and membership information. This makes it possible for any member to easily contact any other member (as-suming they've used their real name) or to e-mail the whole group.
- Members can either send messages via their regular e-mail program or post through the Web site, where they can view the archive of messages and search for a particular message.
- Members can choose their method of message delivery (individual e-mails, daily digests, or access through the Web site) and can access the site features selected by the owner.

If your group decides to use Yahoo Groups, then someone will need to take on the role of group "owner" and go through the process of setting it up. This person need not have a technical background, but it is helpful to have had experience as a member of a similar group. The Web site is http://groups.yahoo.com (look for the comprehensive help section). There are many options in configuring this group, including the opportunity to make it private, available only to those you've invited. Once your group has been set up, you'll invite members to subscribe, and they'll follow Yahoo's directions to do so.

Here are the downsides we found to using the Yahoo Group.

- Some people won't feel comfortable joining a Yahoo Group because of the number of ads they may receive; it's helpful to show them how to opt out of most of the advertising.
- It's not uncommon for people to get lost in the process of trying to subscribe to the group; it's important to provide assistance to these people.
- If this is to be your main method of communication, it's important to encourage everyone in your group to join, or else they'll find themselves out of the loop, and you may not be able to count on this as an avenue for communication.

Being Part of a Group and Sharing the Jobs

CHAPTER TEN

What the Group Means

You've held your first meeting and formed your own unique caregiver family. Your systems are in place, your group's information has been collected and distributed, your lists of captains and co-captains are drawn up, and your group e-mail is working. Part 3 of this book is largely about the jobs caregivers do. But before we discuss the jobs you will do together, let's talk a bit about what it means to be in the group.

Between the time you have your first meeting and the time you feel like a family, you will travel a road with unfamiliar terrain, a lot of bumps, difficult crossroads, and winding detours that seem to go nowhere. But if you let the group have its own special power, it can also be a road with spectacular views, giddy heights, surprises, and miracles.

Journeys You May Take Together

During the life of your caregiver group, you will take many journeys together. But they will not just be journeys to doctors and hospitals. They will be journeys of the heart and mind, journeys of creativity and imagination. One of the journeys we made in Susan's group was to the Bahamas.

About a year before Susan died, the doctors told her there were too many tumors for surgery and that she couldn't take any more radiation. Fighting for her life, she learned of an alternative cancer-treatment program that seemed to have helped a lot of people who were diagnosed as terminally ill, some of whom recovered. It involved close monitoring of the blood and a series of daily injections to boost the immune system so that it could kill the tumors.

The only problem was that the clinic was in the Bahamas, Susan would have to be there for at least six months, and the clinic wouldn't accept her unless she had a full-time companion.

It seemed impossible. We all had jobs, families, responsibilities. But as was usually the case with Susan's group, we would find a way. Cappy volunteered to take Susan to Freeport, enroll her in the clinic, and find a place for her to live. Soon, Joanne volunteered to go with her. Then Susan's daughter Keri said she was coming too.

The group mobilized. Eileen B. spoke with the clinic, arranged for Susan's admittance, and made the travel arrangements. Sheila and Susan's cousin Ferne packed her fourteen suitcases. Eileen M. promised to take care of her apartment. We didn't know how long we could keep her there, but we knew somehow we'd do it.

We checked her into the clinic, found her a beautiful condominium right on the beach, and between regular group members, free-floater members, and Susan's mother, Kay, and sister, Marion, we kept her there for six months. As Cappy recalled:

> It was an amazing journey. We would meet each other at the tiny Caribbean airport as one member would be leaving and another arriving. It was a great comfort for Susan to have people she could really talk to, a large support system, and most of all, hope during this time. Although she was now gravely ill, there were still moments of laughter and friendship and peace. At the clinic, they called us "companions" and the word took on a deep reverence for me. I got to know Susan's daughters and other members of the group in a deeper way. It is a journey I will never forget.

What You May Create Together

Being in a caregiver group isn't always about illness and sad times. It can also be a sharing of joyful times. One of the joyful occasions we created in our group was Susan's daughter's wedding. Susan wanted very much to participate in Elissa's wedding but was very weak at this time. Barbara K., who had a great talent for organization and getting things done, took on the assignment. She found the place, arranged for the ceremony, set the menu, ordered the cake, picked out the flowers, kept track of the costs, and was the driving force that made it happen. But the group pitched in. Cheryl addressed invitations and kept track of the RSVPs, another member arranged for the music, Eileen B. provided a limousine, Sheila did Susan's and the bridal party's makeup, Barbara D. shopped for Susan's dress and jewelry. Susan's brother-in-law, who is a hairdresser, did her hair. Friends and family came from New York and New Jersey, from California and Florida, and Susan, only three months from her death, walked with her ex-husband, Brian, and daughter down the aisle together. This is what Elissa had to say about her wedding day:

> There's one incident about my wedding that makes a particularly good story, as the whole event went perfectly.
>
> Mom's whole Funny Family was there, and I think they can all attest to the fact that Mom was absolutely incredible that day. It was as though she saved up her last reserves of strength and she looked beautiful and healthy. It may have been my wedding, but Mom was truly Queen for a Day, smiling and joyful from start to finish. It was really magical and glorious and I know I will never forget it.
>
> I think that day was her special good-bye to us all, because after it was over, she went into rapid decline and was gone a little over three months later. But she left us all with a really wonderful memory.

Projects You Could Do Together

One group we helped to organize created several projects that turned into major events. Francine, the person the group was taking care of, had been sick with cancer for several years and her finances were severely depleted. But her spirits sank as well when she learned that she needed a bone marrow transplant, an expensive procedure that would require treatment and monitoring for close to a year. That's when her group went into action.

They held a Valentine's dinner dance that raised more than fifteen thousand dollars for Francine's medical costs.

They persuaded various merchants to donate the space, the food, and the services. They got professionals to donate the entertainment. They even had door prizes donated for this charitable event. They advertised the event with flyers and ads in local newspapers and on local radio shows. The cost of the tickets became a tax-deductible item. Everyone in the group participated in this magical Valentine's night . . . a wonderful way to say "I love you" to Francine.

The Valentine Gala was so successful that later, when money was needed again, they held a white elephant sale. All group members, friends, friends of friends—even members of other caregiver groups in the area—donated clothes, knickknacks, furniture, bric-a-brac. It was another true group project. One member collected the items, another got them into presentable shape, another assigned prices. Others were the salespeople, the clean-up crew, the organizers, the accountants.

If there comes a time when you need to raise money for your sick friend, consider a dance, a tag sale, a raffle. Be creative. Enjoy yourself. Spread the jobs among the group members.

Group Problem-Solving

Recognize that group problem-solving is different from individual problem-solving. The whole point of a group is that you don't *have* to do things you don't want to do, are afraid to do, or feel you're not good at. You *can* stop when you're exhausted, you're allowed to be depressed, you *can* cry on someone else's shoulder, you *can* be overwhelmed, you *can* admit to sometimes being a coward, a neurotic, or a jerk (and so can everyone else in the group).

Among all of you is the solution to any problem. Together, you should be able to tackle anything. You don't need to be a therapist, a physician, or a social worker to do some real good. All the tools you need are empathy, common sense, intuition, imagination, communication, and most important of all, the power of the group.

At the beginning, it's important to take the time to get to know the other people, especially the co-captain you've been assigned to work with. When it's your turn to set up the first week, have lunch or a conversation over a cup of coffee with your co-captain and set up the week together. Share your concerns about illness, doctors, hospitals. Be honest about your fears and share your excitement about being part of the group and making new friends.

Making Room for Other People in the Group

If you've been the primary or sole caregiver, and especially if you are a real family member, it may take some doing to adjust to all this new help going toward the person you love, but you will need to address this issue as time goes on or you may end up feeling miserable. For the first four years of her illness, one of the only friends Susan relied on for help was Sheila. After the group was formed and as her illness became worse, she began to single out different people in the group to fulfill her many different needs. When she decided to explore the meaning of her life, she began to work on a screenplay with Cappy about her struggles with cancer and about her group experience. When she needed mothering, she turned to Eileen B., one of the most nurturing and maternal women in the group. This was upsetting to the people who were the closest, especially Sheila, who had been there all along.

As Sheila said:

> Making space for other people became a major adjustment for me. I had always been the first one Susan called on. It made me feel special, needed, and helpful. I recall many a weekend at the beach when she and Cappy would be locked together for hours in deep conversation about the screenplay. I was never invited to participate. It would be a lie to say this never bothered me. Sometimes it made me feel unappreciated and jealous of their closeness. But as time went on, Susan wanted, needed, and demanded to have more of her needs met. It became harder. It was then I began to appreciate all the individual members of the group. I realized that no one person can be "everything" to anyone. The closest we can

come to being everything is to be a "piece of the whole." I learned with the help of the group to do my piece and let the others do theirs.

Letting the Power of the Group Change You

In some magical way that we still don't understand, the group gives everyone exactly what they need. Some people get stronger, more resilient, less afraid. Others get softer, lighter, more willing to go with the flow. The driven workaholic may love being given a job to do and just doing it. The follower may discover his or her leadership qualities. Let your group be an opportunity for you to find new skills, behave differently, explore new sides of yourself. Let the group empower you, support you, heal you.

The following are some thoughts on what Susan's group meant to different people:

> I've never been in a group before. This was a very focused group who had a mission, but that mission embraced us all as we all took care of each other as well as Susan. (T.K.)

> Everyone had one focus—Susan. Everyone cared. Egos were left at home and personal issues were not at hand. (C.R.P.)

> The [group] was a sharing of strength, not of pain and isolation and inadequacy. If I could play sports, it'd probably be like joining a team where everyone could be in the game—nobody was left out. (J.J.)

CHAPTER ELEVEN

The Most Common Caregiver-Group Pitfalls and How to Avoid Them

Ultimately, most people we know who have been in caregiver groups have been moved by the goodness of the human spirit and by the willingness of very different kinds of people to work together. They were surprised at how easily they got to know the strangers in their group, or how much richer their relationships became with the people they already knew. They felt there was very little pettiness, that people tended to be honest and share their true feelings, not criticize each other, and were less selfish than in ordinary circumstances.

But it doesn't just happen. It takes a willingness to work things out together. Every group is different and every group has its own challenges. To help you get off to a good start, here are some of the difficulties that may arise. If they do, remember that all of these pitfalls are human and most of them happen only because everyone is trying to help.

Everyone Is Sure He or She Knows What's Best for the Person Who Is Ill

"She should eat macrobiotic." "She should eat what she wants; she has few enough pleasures." "She should eat my homemade cheesecake." "She should try sushi. After all, the Japanese have a low incidence of cancer." "She should get a second opinion." "She should fire that doctor." "She should meditate." "She should see an acupuncturist." "She should go to church." "She should go to an Indian healer." "She should see a psychiatrist."

What we discovered over three and a half years is that everyone has good ideas and no one knows what's best. One of the most unsettling things about illnesses in the twenty-first century is that in spite of our technological superiority and scientific breakthroughs, even the experts don't have all the answers.

As a member of a caregiver group, your job is to be there for the person who is ill. This means listening, exploring, perhaps researching, talking to doctors, and learning. It means giving the patient permission to try something without judging. Most of all, it means listening to and learning from the rest of the group. *It doesn't mean having all the answers.* No one has them, not even the specialists.

No One Trusts Anyone Else to Do Anything

It is common for each caregiver to feel that he or she is responsible for everything. You don't trust the person who is your co-captain. You're sure he or she isn't up to the job. So you try to control everything that happens in your week. You don't trust the phone chain, so in an emergency you find yourself making all the phone calls. You show up on a night you're not on the schedule just in case the person who is scheduled doesn't.

If you try to do everything, the group won't work. If you don't trust each other, the person who is ill won't trust anyone.

So just do what you said you would do. Show up on Tuesday night. Make your two phone calls. Don't try to do the things you're unsuited for. Don't make judgments about the people in your group. If you follow this advice, you will have many pleasant surprises. The person you thought was a lightweight will turn out to be the calmest person in an emergency you ever met. The person who can hardly get across the room without dropping something, spilling something, or knocking into something will turn out to be the only person the patient trusts to give an injection. The son you were trying to protect may be less afraid than you are.

Crises and emergency situations usually unmask the truth quickly. You may find yourself having a deep, intimate conversation with a complete stranger because you have been thrown together to do something important where your mutual decisions are critical and your cooperation really counts. Just when you thought you'd fall apart, you will find a strength you didn't know was there. You will see people change quickly. There will be less posturing and pretending than in most business or social situations. You may fear that the other person isn't up to the job—and then find out he or she had the same reservations about you.

You may suddenly see that someone else's way of doing something was more efficient or more caring or more logical than yours. Most important, you will see how much we all have in common instead of how different we all are, and you will discover how comforting it is to realize that other people have the same feelings as you.

Everyone Talks about Everyone Else

"I know she can't do this! She can barely take care of herself." "She's so goody-goody. Who does she think she is, Mother Teresa?" "He's always late. What if he doesn't pick her up on time?" "Her eating habits are atrocious. She shouldn't be making her dinner." "Him? If he talks to the surgeon, he'll never get it straight!" "She's so scared. I don't think she can handle this."

If everyone in a caregiver group gives in to gossip, no one will learn to trust anyone else. So if you have a problem with someone in the group, talk to that person directly. Instead of saying "I know she can't handle taking her to the hospital! She can barely take care of herself," say "Sally, I think two of us should go on this one. I think it's going to be a rough trip." Instead of "He's always late," say "Jim, you seem to have trouble showing up on time. Why don't we get someone else scheduled to pick her up from the doctor?"

If you must talk about someone, say something positive. See if you can turn disadvantages into advantages. Use people for what they're good at. Instead of gossiping ("He's so sensitive. I don't think he can handle being there after her chemotherapy"), say "John is so sensitive, he'd be the perfect person to help her when she goes to the physical therapist."

Remember, the more you empower the other people in your group, the eas-ier everything will be on you and your sick friend.

Everyone Filters Everything Through the Person Who Is Ill

This is natural. After all, everyone in the group will know the person who is ill, and many members may not know each other. However, one of the key benefits of a group for the person who is ill is that he or she doesn't have to worry about anything except getting well. Patients don't have to work out schedules, they don't have to ask for help all the time, and they don't have to feel like a burden on one or two people.

If you're not careful, you can create a situation in which the person who is ill is worrying about everyone in the group instead of the other way around. So learn to talk to each other. Have a long phone chat with your co-captain. Go out for lunch or sit down over a cup of coffee. Even if you're complete strangers you already have a common bond. You're there to help someone else. If you've never been part of a team or had to share an impor-tant responsibility, this is an ideal opportunity to learn.

The person who is ill wants your company, your support, your kindness. He or she doesn't want to know all the details, the logistics, and the problems the group is having. Work these things out with the other members of your group.

Everyone Assumes That a Person Who Is Seriously Ill Cannot Contribute to the Group

While you don't want to involve the person who is ill in your group prob-lems or logistics, *you do want to let that person contribute what he or she can.* When Susan quit her job, and before her illness had become too exhaust-ing, there was a long period of time when she discovered (and the group discovered) that she was a great listener. She brought insights to every one of us with her sharp intellect and her practical mind. She also took us on a series of adventures.

[During her struggle] with cancer, Susan read about, learned about, and pursued alternative therapy treatments. There were megadoses of carrot juice, group excursions to the "guru," crystal therapy, and homeopathy. Witnessing the drive, will, and strength of the human spirit was a life lesson [for me]. (D.B.)

So try to have an open mind and overrule your assumptions about people who are sick. You'll be surprised what you may discover. They may learn a new style of cooking and you may learn it with them. They may now be spending a lot of time reading and their conversations may be fascinating. They may even be lighter about life and make you see the value of living in the moment. An evening that started out with bad news may turn into a party as the sick person says he doesn't want to talk about cancer . . . he wants to have a pizza. Then the patient may take you on a series of unexpected adventures as he or she begins to lead a different kind of life.

Everyone Compares What They're Doing to What Everyone Else Is Doing

It cannot be stressed enough! *Every job in a caregiver group is equally important.* Anything you can do is valuable. In Susan's group there were a number of people called "free-floaters." Free-floaters, for various reasons, could not commit to involvement on a weekly basis but were willing to pinch-hit on a job-by-job basis or in an emergency.

No matter how many full-time members you have in your group, there will come a day when a free-floater will be the only one available, will be the relief a burnt-out caregiver needs, or will supply a special skill that no one else has.

Although we had twelve full-time members in Susan's Funny Family, there were a few occasions when free-floaters saved the day. Cappy recalled one such occasion:

Susan had spent the night at my house, debating whether to go to an alternative-care cancer clinic. Her doctor was on the phone telling me she should not be walking around; she should have surgery on her leg. Susan was insisting "No more hospitals, no more surgery!" I was late to a business meeting and Eileen B., who was supposed to relieve me, called and said her back had gone out. I called every regular member I could think of and no one was available until I called Janet, a free-floater, and she said she'd be right over.

When she arrived, I was strung out from fear and exhaustion, Susan was screaming she'd never have surgery again, and Eileen had arrived—bad back and all—with Nicky, her butcher, in tow, carrying a large bag with groceries.

Janet took one look at the three of us and calmly and decisively took charge. She thanked the butcher, took the lunch, filled a hot water bottle for Eileen's back, calmed me down and sent me into the shower, spoke with Susan's doctor, calmed Susan down, and made lunch, all within a half hour of her arrival. She was truly an angel that day.

When you are the captain, don't underestimate your free-floaters. You will find valuable clues in their Individual Data Forms (filled out in the first meeting), and over time you will instinctively know whom to call for what.

The free-floaters in your group are a gold mine of resources. Don't see them as lesser members just because they cannot give the time or full commitment of a regular member.

CHAPTER TWELVE

The Jobs: An Overview

The best way to know your group and to learn to function as a group is to do things together. Try whenever possible to share a job. Work in small teams. Discuss things with each other. Call on other people's skills. When a job is difficult, have three members do it together. When you're afraid, get someone to go with you, and discuss your fears beforehand. If someone offers to do something for *you*, so that you can do something for the person who is ill, accept.

In the next few chapters we have tried to cover most of the major jobs that will come up when taking care of someone with a serious illness. We chose these as examples because we experienced doing them in Susan's group. Your group may have to cope with circumstances not covered here, but seeing how we accomplished our jobs should make it easier to answer your friend's particular needs. Not every job you need to do will be evident at first, and you may discover new jobs along the way. Your group may not always succeed at doing each job perfectly or exactly the way your sick friend might have done it. Someone else may approach a job differently than you. You may learn new skills, do a job you never thought you could do, or learn a better way of doing something from someone else.

To get you going, here is a list of some of the things you can do for a person who is ill. We hope this list will also give you ideas for other tasks your group may want to do. As you can see, even if you had twenty or thirty people in your group, you would find there were enough jobs to go around. You will notice that some jobs are bigger than others. You will discover that no one job is more important than any other.

Jobs Caregivers Can Share

- Give a haircut
- Do the laundry
- Redecorate the patient's room
- Take out the garbage
- Give a pedicure/manicure
- Dust
- Cook dinner
- Take the patient for a drive
- Feed the cat/dog
- Balance the checkbook
- Change the sheets
- Give a massage
- Bring some DVDs or CDs
- Write a Christmas letter, photocopy, and mail it with the patient's Christmas cards
- Give the patient's child a birthday party
- Bring some fresh flowers
- Write a poem
- Transport children to or from school
- "Be there" on Parents' Weekend for the patient's son or daughter
- Set the clocks with the correct time
- Return books to the public library
- Water the plants
- Rake the lawn
- Buy a cheery new bedspread
- Find a terrific nurse's aide
- Find someone to do the patient's taxes
- Help with a shower or bath
- Take the patient away for the weekend
- Put up new curtains in the bathroom
- Do the ironing
- Vacuum the house
- Help a son or daughter with college applications
- Get the newspaper or some magazines
- Bake a cake
- Give a back rub
- Help color the patient's hair
- Walk the dog
- Pick up a package from the post office
- Shovel snow from the driveway
- Start the car when it's below freezing
- Take pictures at a special event
- Make a collage of family photos to hang on the wall
- Visit in the hospital
- Clean the bird cage
- Go to the post office for stamps
- Take the patient out for lunch
- Offer to take the dog for the week
- Help figure out how to handle a problem
- Make a double-dip ice cream cone
- Fill in medical insurance forms ahead of time.
- Write a letter
- Go to the dry cleaner or the drugstore

- Make a nice fruit salad
- Clean the bathroom.
- Get an eyeglass prescription filled
- Take a daughter shopping for her prom dress
- Take a son to camp
- Take a daughter to her dance class every week
- Buy a copy of your favorite bestseller
- Clean out a closet
- Take the patient to chemotherapy appointments
- Find a podiatrist who will make house calls
- Help with putting on makeup
- Take the patient's kids on vacation with your family
- Watch a sports event with the patient
- Program the VCR
- Listen to a fellow group member let out some feelings
- Leave the patient alone when asked to do so
- Help with speech therapy exercises
- Play some soothing music
- Take the kids to their dentist or to a doctor's appointment
- Send the patient's husband off on a fishing trip for the weekend
- Compliment another group member on a job well done
- Take the patient for an astrology reading
- Paint a picture or make an enlargement of a favorite photo
- Celebrate a group member's birthday at the patient's home so he or she won't miss the party
- Write and address thank-you notes
- Send the patient's wife out of town to her sister's for a little R&R
- Take the patient to a dental appointment
- Clear any clutter out of the bedroom

As you begin your jobs, remember that not everything can be done at once; if you try to do too much too soon, you may overwhelm your sick friend or make him or her feel as if you are taking over his or her life. Unless your friend needs total care right away, be careful of coming on too strong. Involve your friend in as many decisions as possible.

Also remember, you've all come together to help someone else. You're all united by a single purpose. No one is getting paid. No one is there to look good. No one will look better if someone else fails. You have a job to do. For many of us, joining Susan's group was the most important job we'd ever been asked to do, and everyone rose to the occasion.

When Your Group Needs to Take On a Big Job

You didn't plan on it or see it coming, but it is possible you will be faced with the challenge of a big job that is of paramount importance to the person who is ill. It might be an issue that affects their income or their safety that needs to be handled pronto. Such a job will test your teamwork, planning, and cooperation, but you will rise to the occasion as a group. That's a lesson these groups learned, when they met—with great success—three very different challenges that couldn't wait.

A Share The Care Group Keeps a Business Running

In New York City, the fifteen members of Shirley's Share The Care Group went beyond their round-the-clock-care duties to keep her retail business operating successfully. That in turn involved the help of others from the community. Melanie describes how their group kept her mother's business running:

> The business was a small flower shop, and yes, it was pretty remarkable that the business continued running since that was *not* the priority for us kids . . . we only cared about making sure Mom was taken care of. But my aunt and uncle (my mom's brother and sister-in-law) had high hopes that my mom would recover and felt the need to keep the business intact for her. So, my uncle would arrive at the shop early each day and place the flower orders to the wholesaler for the day's delivery, and then he'd leave for his job. Then my aunt would arrive and start fulfilling the orders for the day. Of course it helped that she had frequently assisted my mom at the shop in the past so she was very familiar with dealing with customers, making floral arrangements, and so on. Then my aunt recruited some of her retired lady friends and they would take turns each day spending several hours at a time at the store, either running errands, bringing coffee and pastries for coffee breaks, or tidying up the shop and cleaning up at the end of the day. They seem to have created their own impromptu Share The Care for running the business. Each time one of us kids was able to

stop by the store, we were amazed at how organized everything was and at how much money was being collected and deposited into the business account. It was enough to at least cover each month's expenses to keep the business going and to meet payroll . . . and they kept this up for nearly six months, and we only called it quits after my mom passed away.

Looking back now, the only advice I can offer is that if there are factors involved other than caring for the sick person—such as helping to keep a business going, or handling important commitments that the sick person no longer can—just keep in mind that there probably *are* solutions. In my mom's case, all close friends and family were already sharing the care of my mom, so my aunt got the great idea of recruiting store helpers through her pool of friends and community senior citizens center. I believe the women also gained from the experience, being able to feel useful, productive, and appreciated.

Nowadays most people's lives are super busy, but there are good, caring people out there who may have some time and would be willing to volunteer and help. In our case it was the local senior citizens center, but churches, associations, high school and college student organizations also come to mind. I guess it's just a matter of letting people know what you need and asking for the help. Of course when it comes to something like a business, I do advise that the financials be handled by a trusted, responsible person. Other than that, assistance can be sought and found in so many ways.

Taking Care of Summer Rental Property

Keeping another person's life in good working order is a major job, and Cappy's life was no exception. Besides her apartment in New York City, she owned a summerhouse on Long Island. Before she became ill, Cappy had rented her house out (for alternate weekends) to a small group for the summer of 2002. It wouldn't have been in her best interest to cancel the rental when she became ill, because their payments would cover the mortgage costs for the year. So it was imperative to keep this commitment.

Cappy's brother and one person from the Brain Trust took on the summerhouse assignment and made arrangements to get things shipshape for the rental. Having spent time out there, they both knew the inner workings of the house as well as the locals who helped Cappy keep the place in good repair. They opened the house for the season, had it cleaned, shopped for staples, bought a new gas grill, had the water turned on and the gas tanks replenished. They provided the renters, who were new to the house, with important local contact numbers and a guide on how to operate certain things around the house and in the shed. They were the primary contacts for the renters should they need something. At the end of the season they were responsible for getting it cleaned and closed up for the winter.

Moving Out and Into a New House

This information came to us from Barbara, who is part of Jeanie's Share The Care group in Oregon, a cadre of sixteen core members with twenty free-floaters. Though the group just recently formed, as of this writing, they have had to spring into action very quickly. Jeanie was diagnosed with ALS and her physical changes have been rapid. In anticipation of more physical problems down the road, she and her family have had to move into a house with no stairs.

Barbara explains how Jeanie, her husband, and two sons had multiple Share The Care helpers organize the entire move over a period of time.

We had quite a few volunteers that came at different times and worked what they could. Jeanie started off being able to help and orchestrate the beginning process, but gradually she could do less and less. A few weeks before moving, people came over to sort, label, and pack as much as possible. They helped her husband and sons tackle other big jobs like painting the family room, hallway, and stairwell, as well as cleaning, washing carpets, and preparing the house and yard overall for show. (It had not yet been sold.) At the new house another group worked to clean everything before the family's possessions arrived. On moving day, the Share The Care members rented a U-Haul, and about twenty people broke into two groups to handle the move and to put things in storage at another location. (Ten members packed up the truck at the old house and ten others were at the new house waiting to unload.) A team brought food (pizza and beverages) over at lunchtime. It was fortunate that at that time, Jeanie did not require a lot of care other than transportation.

CHAPTER THIRTEEN

Going with Your Friend to the Doctor

One of the most important jobs most group members will do at some point during their friend's illness is to accompany him or her to a doctor or a specialist. It is a job that is often underestimated or overlooked. The person assigned this job must serve as the patient's eyes, ears, and "clear-thinking" mind. Remember, your friend will most likely be in some state of fear or confusion. You must remain sharp and clear. You have to be the calm one and ask the doctor to explain something when you don't understand; you must ask other questions that occur to you during the appointment.

Before the Appointment: Be Prepared

If it is your turn to accompany your friend on a doctor's visit, sit down with him before the appointment and prepare a list of questions he wants to ask (but will forget the moment he gets to the doctor's office) or information he wants to be sure to tell the doctor about his condition. Remember to bring the patient's Central Medical File* binder to the appointment as well as any X-rays or MRIs that might be needed.

Only by asking the doctor a lot of questions can your friend find out all about options for treatment—and possibly relieve some fears by discovering *why* a certain procedure or surgery is needed. During the appointment

* See chapter 15, "Finding Your Way Through the Medical Maze," for more information on this important paperwork.

go through all the questions you have prepared together and write down the answers and specific instructions the doctor gives you. Do not rely on your memory alone to recall such important details.

The questions that come up will, of course, depend on the person's illness and the kind of doctors or specialists being consulted. Following are some possible questions to help get your list going:

- What is this procedure for? Is it routine? Is it to look for something specific?
- What will happen during this procedure?
- How long will the treatment last?
- Does the patient have to do anything special beforehand (for example, no foods or liquids, or drink lots of water)?
- What kinds of reactions might the patient have with this treatment?
- Are there any alternatives to this treatment?
- What is the medication that has been prescribed?
- Will it cause any side effects?
- How does it react with the other medications the patient is taking?
- Please provide information about the specialist who has been recommended.
- How will the patient's life be affected by this illness (surgery, accident)?
- Why is this surgery necessary?
- Will it improve anything?
- What are the risks?
- Will the patient need special care afterward?
- Will he or she need a special diet or exercise?
- What hospital will the patient be going to?
- How long will the patient be there?
- How long will the recuperation period last?

At the Appointment

Now that the two of you are prepared with questions or information for the doctor, arrive promptly for the appointment. Allow extra time for traveling with your friend if he or she has trouble walking or breathing. Take into consideration the weather and traffic conditions. If you think you may need some additional help or know it will be an extremely difficult appointment, ask another member to come with you or ask the captain to find someone who can accompany you.

Note the names of the receptionist and nurse at the doctor's office. Be friendly and try to develop a good relationship with them for your sick friend. They may be helpful to the patient sometime in the future. Help your friend fill out any forms that are needed if he or she doesn't feel well enough to do so (refer to the Medical History and List of Medications, both of which are discussed in chapter 15).

Talking to the Doctor

Your friend will probably be very nervous, so introduce yourself to the doctor and explain that you are part of a caregiver group and have come along to help the patient remember questions, to note what the doctor covers in the appointment, and to ask questions when something is unclear to you or to the patient.

A good attitude is important and will show the doctor that you are serious, responsible, and informed. The doctor will probably be pleased that you and the other members of the caregiver group have taken the time to prepare materials like the Medical History and List of Medications, and will respond to the fact that you are there to help.

After the Appointment

When you have the patient back home, relaxed and comfortable, sit down and go over the things you learned and any doctor's orders he or she will need to follow. If your friend is too tired to discuss the doctor's visit, plan a time to do it as soon as possible. Make copies of any *new* doctor's orders and get them to the captains so other members will be aware of new information. These concerns will also need your prompt attention:

- Notify the captains immediately if any surgery or hospital admittance is to be scheduled, or if the doctor has given the patient any specific orders (i.e., no food or liquids for twelve hours prior to surgery).

- Order and pick up any new prescriptions from the pharmacy as soon as possible.
- When the new prescriptions are picked up, add the drug names to the List of Medications and incorporate the pills into the pillbox for the week. If the patient is taking a considerable number of pills at specific times of day, make sure the new medications are added to the Dosage Schedule.*
- Last, honor your friend's privacy and do not discuss with the group any personal details of this appointment unless the other members need to know them.

* See chapter 15, "Finding Your Way Through the Medical Maze," for information on the List of Medications, creating a pillbox, and the Dosage Schedule.

CHAPTER FOURTEEN

Ten Steps to Making a Hospital Stay as Painless as Possible

Dealing with Hospital Stays

Because Susan had several surgeries, we came to see just how many jobs could be done by the group to make these stressful times easier for everyone. We found there was a lot more we could do than just visit.

We all came to realize not just what Susan needed from us but what we needed from each other, and never did we appreciate our group more. We discovered that most of us had either fears or painful memories or both, and that in the environment of a hospital we were not always at our best. We realized that the sick person is also usually not at his or her best, and we saw how busy and complex hospitals can be.

So we have tried to break down a hospital visit into the following ten steps to help you see the myriad of jobs there are for group members to do and the value of sharing them.

1. Before You Go

- Make arrangements for your friend to go to the hospital comfortably. Have one member with a car drive, or hire a car service or cab. If your friend is in a wheelchair, an ambulette service may be needed. Having the transportation worked out in advance may help to dissipate the person's anxieties (and your friend may well be in a state of "high anxiety").

- If your friend is in the situation that the hospital is going to call when a bed is available (this is not uncommon in larger hospitals), group members assigned must be prepared to move quickly.

- Plan ahead, if possible, for a group member to care for your friend's pets throughout the hospital stay and the recuperation period.
- Don't forget little things like cleaning out perishable items from the refrigerator and emptying the garbage cans. See that plants will be watered by someone every few days and that the house is securely locked.
- In short, do everything you would normally do if your friend was going on a trip. If your friend lives in a house, have several members continue to collect the mail, pay important bills (health insurance and rent),* and pick up the newspapers so the house does not appear empty and an open invitation for a robbery.
- If there is an emergency hospital admission, notify the captains for the week. They will contact real family and start the Telephone Tree to pass information to the group right away. Be sure to give them as many details as possible:

What was the nature of the emergency?
Which hospital was your friend taken to?
Has he or she been admitted?
What is needed?

2. What to Take

- When someone has a serious condition it is always a good idea to keep a small bag packed for an emergency hospital stay. Some of the items that should be included are toothbrush, toothpaste, comb and brush, shaving equipment, glasses, contact lens supply, slippers, robe, pajamas or nightgown. (Note that if you take clothing items you will have to make sure someone takes them home to be laundered—hospitals don't do this—and replaces them with fresh ones.) If the patient wants to take other clothes, make sure they are easy to get in and out of—no tight waistbands or complicated buttons. Leave all valuables at home. This means jewelry, watches, and rings. (If the patient is to have surgery he or she cannot wear any of these items into the operating

---

* See chapter 20, "Getting Their Affairs in Order," for more information.

room, and the hospital is not responsible for any valuables you take in.) Don't take any large amounts of cash—take just enough to purchase a magazine or other small items on the hospital shopping cart (usually candy, cookies, toys, magazines, papers, and so on). A group member can be assigned the job of holding the cash and paying for the patient's TV and phone.

- Take all medications with you. Even though hospitals legally need to dispense medications from their own pharmacy through their own personnel, the pill-box is a great help to make sure the sick person doesn't miss any pills while waiting to be processed into a room. This is especially important if the time when the medication is taken is critical. Have a copy of the List of Medications and the Dosage Schedule so the medical staff is aware of everything the patient is taking.

- Take the Central Medical File binder or a copy of the Medical History* with you. Also be sure to bring insurance cards and numbers, and copies of the Living Will and Health Care Proxy† for their files. Know which doctor ordered the hospital stay or surgery so you can refer to him if necessary.

- Take the patient's personal address/phone book.

- Take a copy of the Share The Care Yellow Pages.

- Take some things for your friend's personal entertainment: a book, magazines, a pack of cards, knitting, an inexpensive CD player and CDs, and so forth. Also remember your friend's rosary, Bible, or prayer book if these things are important to him or her.

- Take an inexpensive vase. It is amazing how difficult it can be to locate a vase in a hospital.

- Take something silly and cheery like a favorite teddy bear (even for grown-ups).

- If the patient arrives with the help of his or her own walker, cane, or wheelchair, be prepared to take it back to his or her home until he or she is discharged. The hospital will supply one if needed, and any personal item like this may be lost.

---

* See chapter 15, "Finding Your Way Through the Medical Maze," for information on the List of Medications, Dosage Schedule, Medical History, and Central Medical File.
† See chapter 20, "Getting Their Affairs in Order," for information on the Living Will and Health Care Proxy.

3. Accompanying the Patient

Make sure two group members are assigned to accompany the sick person to the hospital or emergency room: one to deal with the logistics, one to be with the patient. This point cannot be stressed enough. Entering a hospital is a scary, off-putting experience for most people. You will encounter other patients, hospital personnel rushing about, and odd smells and sounds. You may pass someone being resuscitated, or hear someone screaming. There is so much to deal with that one caregiver cannot take care of the logistics and take care of the person who is being admitted at the same time, especially if your friend is very nervous or very ill.

If you, personally, have a problem just being in a hospital, do not volunteer for this job. If you have been assigned the job, call the captain and request another job (feed your friend's cat, clean up and secure the home, or make needed phone calls). Have the captains find another member who is more relaxed about going to hospitals and following through.

4. Admitting the Patient

Be prepared to wait, to try two different buildings before you find the right one, to tell the patient's medical history several times, to fill out forms, to run around to several floors, to fill out more forms, and (especially in a city hospital) to get lost. The medical establishment and the hospital system are run by human beings, and just like workers in any business, these people are overworked, overbooked, and sometimes overwhelmed.

Be sure that the copies of the patient's Living Will and Health Care Proxy go into the hospital file upon admittance (the doctor should also know about these important documents ahead of time and have copies in his own files). Check with the nurses on the floor after your friend has been admitted and settled into a room to make sure these papers are in the file and that the medical staff are aware of them.

5. Working with Hospital Personnel

There is a way to work with doctors and other hospital personnel that will make everything easier for your loved one, your group, and them. Taking some responsibility (by bringing the patient's Medical History and List of Medications, for instance) is a good way to begin. Remembering what they tell you is an important next step (write everything down and pass along the information to other members). Having one member to keep the patient calm while another member talks to the hospital staff can help everyone.

Also keep track of all the "angels" you run across . . . the receptionist who's always friendly and helpful, the driver of the ambulette service who's always patient, and the hospital orderly who always waters your friend's plants when he comes in to mop the floor. Keep a list of these people so you and the other members can call them by name, thank them, and acknowledge them. They are also honorary and valuable members of your caregiver group, and if you treat them kindly they will remain helpful.

When the patient has been settled into a room a nurse will come in to get all the important information that might have been overlooked in Admitting. This is where having copies of the patient's Medical History and List of Medications will be of value. As a caregiver, you can be helpful to the nurse in covering all important information if your friend is nervous or not feeling well. Be sure to identify to the nurse any special conditions the patient may have—he or she can't hear very well and won't use a hearing aid, he or she is confused much of the time, he or she wears glasses or contact lenses or has a full set of dentures.

6. Getting Settled in the Room

When your friend is assigned a room, one of you should make some quick checks to see if he or she has everything needed. Is the temperature comfortable? Is there enough air-conditioning or too much heat? Are the lights working? Is there a buzzer for the nurse? Does your friend have a roommate?

On one occasion when we checked Susan into the hospital, she was assigned to a room with an elderly lady who would not stop screaming. Susan became nearly hysterical at the prospect of remaining in the room and threatened to leave that minute if she didn't get another one, despite the fact that she was scheduled for important surgery the next day. One of us did a quick survey of the floor—while the other stayed with Susan—and discovered that there was, in fact, another room much farther down the hall that was available. We were able to have her moved when we calmly and very politely (yet firmly) suggested this solution to the head nurse.

7. Getting Connected

Now that a room has been secured, the next job is to get the TV set up and paid for and the phone hooked up. (Most hospitals charge additional fees for these services.) While one person handles that, another member can take notes for the group regarding visiting hours, the room number and floor, the phone number, and the general situation. One of you can then make a call to one of the captains so they can get this information out to all the members via e-mail or telephone and schedule various visiting times on their weekly Caring Schedules. Also include any information you can get from the head nurse about the patient's surgery (if that is the reason for the hospital stay). When is it scheduled? How long will it take? How long will your friend be in the recovery room? What would be a good time for a fellow caregiver to be here?

If your friend is admitted to an intensive care unit (ICU), special rules and visiting times will have to be followed. For example, sometimes a visitor, usually only family, can visit in an ICU for only fifteen minutes at a time. If your friend has no family and your caregiver group is his or her only support, you may have to explain the situation to the doctor or the head nurse to get some sort of special permission so members may visit at scheduled times. Be aware that group members who are particularly squeamish or fearful of hospitals may not wish to visit a friend in an ICU. These special units are usually filled with several seriously ill patients who are hooked up to machines and life-support systems.

8. Being with Your Friend in the Hospital

Being There When He or She Wakes Up

Just being hospitalized can be quite frightening. Having surgery can really cause great anxiety in your friend. It is a great relief to a patient to see a friendly face there when being brought back to the room from recovery. Even though the person will be groggy or very tired and probably not up to talking, just knowing you are there will be very reassuring. Captains will have to arrange for this very important first visit, and it is up to you, if you are assigned, to be there on time.

> Actually Susan's fear of surgery and hospitals required only one thing: To know she was not alone and someone she trusted was there to stand guard. (W.F.)

Making Your Friend's Stay More Comfortable

When you visit, you can always bring flowers, special foods (if allowed), mail (forget the bills and junk mail; bring what looks like letters or cards), a cute toy, fruit, balloons, or even just your smiling face. You can help your friend by combing his or her hair or getting the water pitcher refilled. Find out from the nurse's aides where you can do this. Some hospitals even have microwaves so you can heat something up for your friend. Run down to the hospital store for more tissues or other sundries.

Sheila recalls an unusual incident that happened during one of Susan's hospital stays:

> Susan loved stone crabs from a particular restaurant in Miami, and when Cappy was in Florida, she found they would send orders out by air to New York. When I arrived for my evening visit to Susan with the crab legs and mustard sauce and my trusty little hammer, I thought she would go nuts. I couldn't crack and peel those little suckers fast enough for her. She was in absolute heaven and God only knows what the people in the next room thought. We were pounding with the hammer and squealing in delight as she finished off what she described as "the finest meal" she ever enjoyed in a hospital.

Bring your friend up-to-date on what's happening at home. Are you staying with the children? Are you watching a pet for your friend? Help your friend go for a walk around the halls of the hospital. Put a ribbon in her hair.

There are so many things you can do to make a hospital stay easier. It's a good idea to get to know the nursing staff while your friend is in the hospital. Be friendly—you can accomplish more this way. Learn the names of as many of the nurses and nurse's aides as possible.

It is also a nice gesture to give the staff some candy or cookies and a thank-you card from your friend. Captains take note, and don't forget to assign a member this job. It is conceivable the patient could come back to the same hospital and have the very same people taking care of her at a later date. People remember being thanked for their efforts and may go out of their way just a little bit more to help your friend.

9. Dealing with Health Insurance— Don't Forget to Follow the Rules

If the patient's hospital stay was planned, make sure the member assigned to this area notifies the medical health insurance* advocate in advance. If surgery is involved, a second doctor's opinion was probably required. If a hospital admittance was an emergency, it is very important that the group member responsible contact the insurance company as soon as possible. Be familiar with the policies of the individual insurance company beforehand and know the procedures that need to be followed. It could be financially catastrophic if you fail to do this.

10. Creating a Pleasant Homecoming

It's always nice to come home after a long hospital stay . . . especially when your home is fresh and inviting.

Captains should have a couple of members air out the house or apart-

---

* See chapter 20, "Getting Their Affairs in Order," for important details on health insurance forms and procedures.

ment and straighten things up before your friend comes home. It's a loving touch to have some cheery flowers on the table and at the bedside and clean linens on the bed.

Before your friend leaves the hospital, have one of the members check to see if there are any special dietary instructions for the patient. The hospital dietician may supply a list of foods your friend may eat. Make sure the group is aware of any food restrictions so they don't show up with a major temptation your friend won't be able to enjoy. If it is a soft-foods diet the captains will need to have someone make flavored gelatin or a light custard. They will have to make sure to have sherbet and juices on hand too. If no special diet is required the refrigerator should be restocked with staples: milk, juice, soda, bread, and so forth.

Captains should assign a "fresh" member to take over from the members who brought the patient home from the hospital. These members may have to go back to work or may just be exhausted. Don't overlook the possibility that it could be very hard for your friend to suddenly be left alone after having the hospital staff looking in on her constantly. She may need a lot of extra tender loving care for a while. Or, on the other hand, your friend may be looking forward to the peace and quiet of her own home, and captains should be aware not to overload the schedule with a lot of visitors.

CHAPTER FIFTEEN

Finding Your Way Through the Medical Maze

Sitting with Susan in doctors' offices and listening to her many tales of hospitalizations, surgeries, and radiation treatments made all of us realize how hard it was for her to repeat these painful experiences and how easy it might be to forget something or confuse the order of these procedures or their dates.

Chances are, the person your group is helping is taking a lot of medications too. Are they for pain? How often do they have to be taken? Are there specific instructions—take before bedtime or take on an empty stomach? As caregivers you may need to know this information at some point.

It occurred to us that a central file containing all this information would save the patient endless and often painful reporting of his or her medical history and would give new specialists, doctors, and therapists a complete and quick overview of the case. Most important, it would allow any group member to give accurate information if the patient was confused or unconscious at the time it was needed.

Other groups have found having a central file very valuable. Sometimes information has been scattered. Different doctors have been affiliated with different hospitals. Patients have had treatments in another city. A key administrative person who had been keeping track of everything is no longer there. With the complexity of modern medical treatment and with so many medical personnel being overburdened, don't expect them to keep track of the records of your loved one. Let the group do it.

Finding the Right Team

Captains could ask for two committed and detail-oriented group members to volunteer for the very important responsibility of organizing the patient's medical information and continually keeping it up-to-date.

If two members work on this job together it will be less likely that an important detail (which might make a huge difference to a doctor) will be overlooked.

Creating a Central Medical File

If you are on the team that has elected to do this job you will be collecting information for the following charts:

Medical History chart (see page 177)
List of Medications chart (see pages 182–83)
Dosage Schedule (if needed; see page 187)

Also to be included in the Central Medical File will be copies of the patient's medical directives (Living Will, Health Care Proxy.) * These documents may or may not have been completed by the patient at the time you are compiling the Medical File. If they are done, be sure to include several photocopies. If not, keep checking with the group members who are helping the patient get his or her affairs in order.

Download the charts we've provided and make several copies of each in case you need extras. You can also create your own versions to suit the patient's specific case, especially if it is very long or complicated.

We recommend you purchase a large (2"–3" thick), bright (so you can easily locate it) loose-leaf binder and add dividers for different sections: Medical History, Medications charts, Dosage Schedule, Medical Directives, Hospital Discharge Instructions, the Weekly Schedule, and Daily Observations. Purchase lots of 3-hole lined paper as well for the Daily

---

* See chapter 20, "Getting Their Affairs in Order," for information on completing these important legal documents.

Observations. If you purchase a loose-leaf book with a clear plastic open-ing on top you can slide a sheet of paper in the front with this label:

Name   's

CENTRAL MEDICAL FILE
Medical History
Medications Charts
Dosage Schedule
Medical Directives
Hospital Discharge Instructions
Weekly Schedule
Daily Observations*

On the first page of the binder or on the inside of the plastic cover add the following information about the patient:

Name:
Address:
Telephone:
Date of Birth:
Allergies:

Collecting the Medical History

Next you will need to schedule some time with the patient to go over his or her medical history. We suggest two hours for this part so no one feels rushed.

Then, with the patient's help and the use of his or her address book, e-mail address list, Palm Pilot, Rolodex, date books, and calendars—as well as his or her copies of medical insurance claim forms—start clearly listing the following in order of their occurrence:

---

* If you prefer, you could put the Weekly Schedule and Daily Observations in a separate loose-leaf binder in a different color (this one should definitely be 3" thick).

- Date of illness
- Diagnosis
- Physician or specialist (include telephone and address)
- Type of treatment (therapies, radiation, chemotherapy, surgery); include names of surgeon, radiologist
- Date of surgery, treatment, or therapy
- Hospital where treated

Also, collect any other information or papers that seem like they should be part of this record and add them to the file. These could include copies of surgeon's postoperative reports, copies of X rays, or copies of MRIs. Store X rays, MRIs, and other large film records in their original envelopes, with dates, in a special cool place away from sunlight where they will not be damaged.

As the illness progresses or if the patient has a long medical history already, you may find the charts are not big enough to include all the information. Then we suggest you create a long-form medical history on the computer that tracks all the pertinent information. (An example is on pages 178–80.) This document can be easily updated as the illness progresses. Write short paragraphs, by date, describing relevant details of what occurred or what treatments were received. At the top of the chart include information such as name, address, telephone, date of birth, Social Security, insurance information, family history, allergies, and who to call and telephone numbers in case of an emergency. It can be a life-saving document for a very ill patient to carry whenever going out.

After reconstructing this medical history, particularly if it is long and complicated, the patient may feel too tired to discuss medications. If so, you will have to schedule another hour for this. Do it as soon as possible.

Name: _____
Address: _____
_____

Date: _____

SHARE THE CARE
MEDICAL HISTORY

DATE OF ILLNESS	DIAGNOSIS	PHYSICIAN/SPECIALIST	TYPE OF TREATMENT	DATE OF SURGERY	HOSPITAL

SAMPLE OF LONG-FORM MEDICAL HISTORY

Name:

Address:

Telephone:

Date of birth:

SS#:

Insurance information and group number:

Carry With You
Medications/water
Yellow pages/cell phone
Insurance card:
Picture identification

Allergies:

Prior illnesses:

Prior surgeries:

Family history:

Current medications:

Person(s) to notify in case of an emergency:

Name	Telephone #'s
1.	
2.	
3.	

History of illness, including surgeries and treatments: (Include list of all hospital and doctors' names/addresses and telephone numbers on separate sheet.)

2 wks. prior	Complaints of difficulty getting words out. Attributed to stress.
3/14/02	First experience of numbness to the face. Emergency Medical Service called, taken to Example Hospital, Orange County. CAT scan showed a mass on brain. Dr. One.
3/26	At Example Medical Center in New York biopsy confirms diagnosis of Grade IV Glioblastoma located on left side near Broca's Center. Patient declined chemotherapy and radiation therapy. Surgeon is Dr. Two.

4/01	Began alternative treatment with Doctor Three in Florida.
4/14	Suspended alternative treatment and went to Boston for neurosurgery. Speech difficulty increasing.
5/19	Neurosurgery at Example Hospital. Dr. Four. Successful debulking of approximately 80% of tumor mass. Lost fine motor skills in right hand. Lost remaining ability to speak. (Both slowly returning with physical and speech therapy.)
6/21	Went to Example Hospital ER in New York complaining of shortness of breath in chest. Diagnosed with PCP pneumonia, blood clots in lungs and leg by Dr. Five. Filter inserted through groin area to help keep clots from going to brain by Dr. Six. Sixteen days in hospital.
7/16	Released from hospital. Home treatment for PCP pneumonia.
7/17	Follow-up appt. with Dr. Five. PCP pneumonia responding well to treatment.

Overall, patient continues to have difficulty speaking and writing—combination of surgical procedure and tumor location. Patient continues to be on medications (see list) to control seizures and steroids to reduce tumor swelling. Patient has had six "episodes" similar to original event (numbness on right side of face, loss of right-hand motor skills) that last approximately 30 minutes.

9/24	Patient resumed treatment at Florida clinic yet never settled into a steady regimen and constantly had difficulty staying on the treatment.
9/21	Emergency intestinal surgery at Example Medical Center, Florida. After complaining about stomach pains for approximately one week, patient was given an MRI, where they discovered a tear in colon. Dr. Six.
9/23	Since the surgery and probably as a result of the anesthesia, patient has had a significant weakening on right side

and cannot now use right hand or right leg. The edema continues.

Before surgery, after having an ultrasound, Dr. Seven said liver was slightly enlarged. On September 30 the clinic discontinued the treatment until patient came back to NY, and tests show that liver enzymes have come down.

Doctors and hospital names and addresses are attached. Current list of medications schedule is also attached.

Getting Medications Organized

Organizing your friend's medications will make a positive difference that can be appreciated by the patient and other caregivers right away. At the end of this chapter there are also some specific tips on how to organize medications for the week and help your friend remember to take them at specific times.

For this stage, find a basket, tray, or box that is big enough to hold all the patient's medications; keep it in one central place where all of the caregivers can easily locate it. There may be exceptions; for example, certain drugs need to be refrigerated or frozen. Keep them in special containers that have been clearly labeled, and put a note on the refrigerator door to remind others that medications are stored inside, and to be careful about moving or accidentally throwing them away.

While you have all the medications together, go over the following list:

- Get rid of all medications that are past their expiration dates and confirm with the physician that they need not be refilled.
- If the patient can no longer remember what the medication is for, check with the physician. The medication may no longer be necessary.
- Keep all medications out of the reach of small children.

Filling Out the List of Medications

Sitting together with the patient, review all his or her pills, liquids, drops, shots, or sprays while another member of your team carefully fills in all the information listed on the chart for each drug:

- Name of medication and Rx number
- Refills
- Dosage
- Physician
- What is it for?
- Special instructions

The List of Medications proved to be a crucial piece of information when Susan was very ill and one of our members had to call her doctor in the middle of the night. It was a big help having all the information and actual medications at hand so the caregiver was able to tell the doctor what Susan had available and he was able to prescribe something to relieve her problem. See List of Medications chart on pages 182–183.

Keep an Observation Journal

Taking a tip from medical professionals, who are required to keep records of the patient's vital signs, it is a good idea to start a daily Observation Journal. This can be kept in a section of the Central Medical File binder or, if you prefer, as a separate binder along with the Weekly Schedule. This kind of information will be especially helpful in cases when the patient's condition is subject to changes in mood, appetite, or physical abilities that need to be reported back to the physician. The Observation Journal is the responsibility of each visiting caregiver. Make sure all of the group members read about this job carefully and are diligent about keeping it going.

Some of the following guidelines for keeping the Journal were submitted by Dotty, who has worked with seriously ill patients for years.

- Date each page and have it filled out by caregivers as they change shifts (list their name and hours spent with patient).

SHARE THE CARE **LIST OF MEDICATIONS**		Pharmacy Name: _____ Tel: _____ Address: _____		

Name: _____
Address: _____
_____
Telephone: _____
Date of Birth: _____

ALLERGIES:

Refills	Name of medication and Rx#	Dosage	Physician	What's it for? Special instructions
1 2 3 4 5				
1 2 3 4 5				
1 2 3 4 5				
1 2 3 4 5				

LIST OF MEDICATIONS

Refills	Name of Medication and RX#	Dosage	Physician	What's it for? Special instructions
1 2 3 4 5				
1 2 3 4 5				
1 2 3 4 5				
1 2 3 4 5				
1 2 3 4 5				

- The Journal can contain all kinds of information: how long the patient slept, what they ate (including what/how much they ate or drank), how they were feeling (tired, agitated, upset), what time they actually took their meds.
- If any problems came up, report how they were solved. One could also log any telephone calls that came in. This information will be very helpful to the next person who comes for their shift if there isn't enough time to go into detail about the day.
- Please print so that it will be easy to read by all. Make the information brief and factual. It is something that can be read by the person who is ill or any of their caregivers. Keep it near the bed for easy location.

A Feelings Journal

A Feelings Journal is optional but quite valuable. If caregivers or the patient wish to record their personal feelings, inspirations, or discoveries, keep these in a separate section in the binder (if it is a loose leaf with sections) or a separate Feelings Journal. It may turn out to be a revealing record of how the group and patient were doing emotionally. It is an excellent way to recognize and release many of our pent-up responses. The group can also learn that others share their same fears, worries, and anxieties. Our vulnerabilities can then bring us closer. When we share some of our feelings with the person who is ill, they may be less likely to think that anyone is talking behind their back. Several groups have commented that they found such journals to be very therapeutic for everyone.

Keeping the Information Current

When the Medical History, Medications Chart, and Dosage Schedule are completed, make several copies and put them in a pocket in the binder to leave one behind, if needed, at a doctor's office or hospital. Also, make several copies of Medical Directives for the same purpose. Depending on the complexity of your loved one's illness, you could take the complete Central Medical File binder with you to an appointment (keep it in its own special bright canvas bag so it is not left behind or lost), or just bring current copies of the above-mentioned information.

If you volunteered to be a member of the team for the Central Medical File information, be vigilant about keeping it current. Make sure it is updated after every doctor visit, and add or delete medications as appropriate. Though this can be handled by the group member who accompanies the patient to the doctor's appointment,* it is still up to the team to check to see that it was done and to continually keep the binder neat.

Note: The Central Medical File is vital and should always be kept in one specific place in the patient's home (perhaps with the medications basket or box, at the bedside, or next to the telephone). Be sure to notify every group member, as well as the family and free-floaters, of its existence, purpose, and exact location so that it can be found easily in the event of an emergency.

Three Foolproof Ways to Help Your Friend with His or Her Medications

1. The Pillbox

Dealing with Susan's many different medications became so complex that we created our own specialized pillbox for her. Since then, the pillbox has worked for a number of people.

* See chapter 13, "Going with Your Friend to the Doctor," for more information on caregivers' responsibilities.

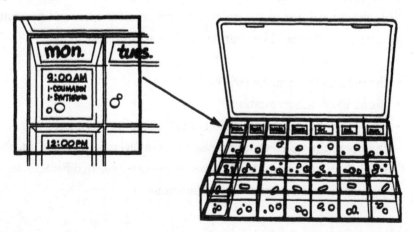

Purchase a clear plastic box with small compartments. Ideally, it will have seven compartments across the top (one for each day of the week) and four or five compartments down (depending on the number of times pills will need to be taken). You can find these boxes in hardware, sporting goods, or variety stores.

Next, with adhesive tape and a permanent Magic Marker, label the days of the week across the back (top) row. Then cut out small squares of paper (to fit each compartment down the left side) and label each one with the name of the medication and the time of day it is to be taken (see illustrations on page 185). By putting this information on small squares of paper, it can easily be replaced or changed if medication changes are ordered by the doctor. You can read down and across and see instantly what needs to be taken or if it has been taken.

Now the box is ready to be filled with all the medications needed for the entire week. Your friend will not have to open countless pill bottles every day or try to remember if he or she took the five o'clock pills.

There are also numerous pillboxes sold in pharmacies that can be used if you feel you don't need to create your own version.

2. The Dosage Schedule

If your friend is taking vast quantities of medications and vitamins throughout the day, we suggest you create a simple Dosage Schedule on the computer so it can be updated weekly and then saved as a record in a binder. (See the sample Dosage Schedule on page 187.) Though this means a little more work for someone, it will save precious time and prevent any mix-ups or confusion. The chart should clearly indicate

- the week that the schedule will be in effect
- the name of each medication
- what time of day each medication needs to be taken
- the size of the tablet, usually measured in milligrams (mg); *pay attention* to this information on the bottle as medicines can come in different sizes and a mistake on number or size can be disastrous

SAMPLE DOSAGE SCHEDULE FOR : JUNE 7 THROUGH JUNE 13		
6:00 am		Decadron 3 mg (0.75 mg. X 4) Protonix 40 mg.
6:45 am		Bromelain (3)
7:00 am	**WITH BREAKFAST**	DHEA 100 mg Boswellia (3) Vitamin (1) Berberine sulfate (1) Vitamin E (1) Tonic in beverage, 3 dropperfuls
8:00 am		Keppra 1000 mg Fish oil 3 teaspoons
11:00 am		Decadron 0.75 mg
12:00	**WITH LUNCH**	Vitamin (1) Vitamin E (1) Berberine Sulfate (1) Advacal (2) Boswellia (3) Tonic in beverage, 3 dropperfuls Bactrim (1) Celebrex 100 mg
2:00 pm		Boswellia (3) Bromelain (3)
4:00 pm		Celebrex 100 mg
7:00 pm	**WITH DINNER**	Vitamin (1) Vitamin E (1) Berberine sulfate (1) Advacal (2) Boswellia (3) Tonic in beverage, 3 dropperfuls
8:00 pm		Celebrex 200 mg Thymus 4 sprays Bromelain (2)
9:00 pm		Homeopathic treatment (yellow)
10:00 pm		Gingko (2) Keppra 1000 mg HCT 25 mg Klor-Con (1)
10:30 pm		Metatonin 20mg Zinc (1)

- number of pills to be taken based on mg. size
- special instructions (take with food or take with water only)

3. The Timer

When someone has a lot of medications to take throughout the day it is a good idea to have a reminder. Buy a kitchen timer that the patient can keep nearby throughout the day and take along whenever he or she leaves the house.

Doing Personal Things for Your Friend

There may come a point in your friend's illness when some very personal jobs need to be done. You may be asked to empty a portable toilet, help your friend take a shower, or buy special undergarments for incontinence.

Certain members within the group may feel less inhibited and more capable of doing these kinds of things, and the captains should try to assign them these jobs whenever possible. But if, in an emergency, you are called upon to do something personal (and you feel somewhat surprised, shocked, or fearful) and there is no one else to do it . . . do the best you can do.

It may help to remember that the person who is ill may also be embarrassed by the situation. Your friend may become upset and cry. He or she may get angry and frustrated. Let your friend express these feelings. Don't pretend these feelings don't exist. Acknowledge them—whether with a hug, a touch, or an understanding word.

Special Medical Equipment

At some point, someone who is ill or elderly may become unsteady on his or her feet and need a cane or walker to get around. And in some cases, if this condition worsens, such a person may need a wheelchair.

Susan felt strange when she started to need the help of a cane. But she came to discover a real benefit (besides the support it gave) from having one. Whenever she went out on the streets of New York City, having a cane was a "signal" to people to give her some space or to be a little more polite. Once she realized this she would go nowhere without it.

As the caregivers for a sick, elderly, or injured friend, you will discover the huge assortment of medical equipment, supplies, gadgets, and special furniture to help people be more secure and comfortable in their home. The Internet is full of information on a variety of products, from power chairs to lifts to ramps and toilets that can wash and dry a person after use (made by Neorest, a Japanese company, and very expensive). For a wide variety of products, equipment, and discounts check out The Caregivers Marketplace at http://www.caregiversmarketplace.com.

The Spinal Cord Injury Information Network at http://www .spinalcord.uab.edu is one of the most comprehensive Web sites we have found. It provides a wide range of current information on all areas of coping with physical problems, not just spinal injuries. If you assign a team to explore the Internet for solutions, this is a great place to start checking out some of the following areas: accessibility issues; clothing solutions for a wide variety of problems; car/van modifications; equipment and medical supplies; ramps; and much, much more.

The team can also call local hospitals, medical equipment stores (where long-term or short-term rentals can also be applied to purchase), and pharmacy sections of large drugstores in your community. Also check senior citizens centers, as they often have a loaner bank of equipment. You may find some secondhand equipment in very good condition at rummage sales, flea markets, and thrift stores for a reasonable price and big savings.

Expensive Equipment

Before investing in very expensive equipment (hospital beds, wheelchairs) there are several things to take into consideration:

1. Check with the patient's doctor or physical therapist about *what* to rent or purchase. Please note: When a doctor orders special equipment (that is, when it is *prescribed*), it becomes a deductible item for many health-care plans. Be sure to have the group member in charge of the medical insurance area check to see if the cost of a specific item is covered.
2. The insurance provider that pays for the equipment may require that you

purchase from specific suppliers. Ask about this before you spend a lot of time searching—or worse yet, rush into an unreimbursable purchase.

3. Be sure of what your sick friend needs and wants.

If the members of the group enjoy taking your friend out to the mall, to lunch, or to a special event, but find that the patient has difficulty walking even short distances, has problems breathing, or tires very easily, consider the purchase of a very lightweight folding wheelchair. It can be picked up, packed into a car trunk by even the smallest member of your group, and is a terrific solution to keeping the patient involved in social activities as long as possible.

If the patient is bedridden, an electric hospital bed (that can be raised and lowered, and is equipped with bedrails) could be the very best solution for his or her comfort as well as a saving grace for the caregivers' backs.

Keep in mind that equipment can cause anxiety for people who already feel helpless. When Sheila's mom needed a wheelchair, Sheila thought a motorized one would be great. However, when her mom tried it, she was terrified that she wouldn't be able to stop it. For her, the normal wheelchair turned out to be a better idea.

Before you put someone in a wheelchair, it might be a good idea to take a ride in one yourself. Discover how it feels when the chair comes to a sudden halt and you feel like you will go flying out of it. Experience the sensation of hitting a sudden bump, and how vulnerable it feels to have your feet sticking out. You will discover that it can be very unsettling until you get used to it—and you will have more compassion for the person you are wheeling.

Equipment and Gadgets That Make Things Easier

If the bathroom is located down a hallway from your sick friend's bedroom and he or she is in any way unsteady, has bad eyesight, or is easily disoriented at night, purchasing a portable toilet to keep at the bedside could relieve a feeling of panic for the patient.

As you will see in the next section, there are numerous things that can be purchased to assist your friend. However, if money is an issue, your group may want to brainstorm for ways of creating solutions without spending a great deal. We encourage you to use your imaginations, experience, and individual talents, as there may be three or four new ways to solve a problem.

Suppose your friend is getting terribly frustrated because she needs the use of a walker and is constantly having to ask for assistance in doing even the smallest task (like transporting a book or magazine across the room). Attach a small bicycle basket to the front of the walker with some wire so she can do some things without any assistance.

If there is a nightstand or desk filled with items (remote controls, pillbox, phone, etc.) and your friend is having difficulty reaching things, put these items on a large plastic lazy Susan so they can be reached when needed without a lot of effort.

What Kinds of Equipment and Gadgets Are Available?

Here is a sampling of some of the products available to help your sick friend. See what might apply to his or her particular case and get out there and find it.

- Portable ramps for wheelchairs
- Practical clothing with snap-back closures
- Pads, pillows, special bedding
- Walkers with wheels/baskets/seats
- Audio solutions for rest and relaxation
- Armchairs with controls to recline to an almost bed position and a lift mechanism to bring the patient to a standing position
- Grippers for picking things up off the floor
- Disposable underpads and sheeting for the bed
- Special supports for men and women (back, abdomen, hernia, etc.)
- Elevated toilet seats
- Swivel cushions for getting in and out of a car
- Blood pressure monitors
- Grab bars and rails for bath and shower
- Bath seats or benches

- Portable lifts
- Portable toilets
- Digital thermometers
- Specialized fitness equipment
- Arm and leg exercises for people in wheelchairs
- Shampoo rinse trays for washing hair in sink while seated
- Wheelchair trays
- Disposable incontinence products
- Rolling tables
- Special mattress pads to reduce pressure, give extra support and comfort, and improve circulation for bedridden patients
- Walker with seat—to sit and rest in between walking
- Wireless intercom/baby room monitor
- "The Clapper"—an electronic device that turns appliances on and off by clapping
- Boards for assisting moves from bed to wheelchair

CHAPTER SIXTEEN

Caregiving at Home (and Far from Home)

Caregiving at Home

Knowing What the Group Shouldn't Do

Think for a minute about what it would be like to be seriously ill or disabled and have a group of people who didn't know what they were doing try to help you. It would be frightening.

Never pretend to know what you are doing when dealing with someone's physical care (lifting or moving, getting a patient in and out of a wheelchair and into a bed, changing bed linens while the patient is in bed, or even assisting them to walk). If some members of the group try to do some of these jobs without training or knowledge, they could easily injure the patient as well as themselves.

Where the Group Can Get Special Training, If Needed

Should the patient be totally bedridden and group members volunteer to take on some of the home-care jobs, they will need to learn some new skills. Many of the important daily physical tasks needed are easy to do once you have been taught the correct way to do them.

An interested member can volunteer to contact the patient's physician, the hospital social worker, or the local Department of Social Services or senior citizens center to find out where group members can get home-care instruction. Another important source of help would be the organization that deals with your loved one's specific illness. For example, your local ALS association can help with special training and skills for caregivers of ALS patients. Additional or special training and precautions must also be sought if members are to give injections, deal with feeding tubes, or care for someone in an advanced stage of AIDS. Group members may also want to consider a course in first aid or CPR. This knowledge may be of great value at another time in your lives, as well. See the list of Helpful Associations at the back of this book for contact information.

Getting the Professional Help You Need

It is also possible your group may be faced with a situation where total home care is suddenly needed (for example, accident, surgery, or stroke). If this is the case, have a team of group members get assistance and information about agencies from the hospital staff and doctor *before* the patient is sent home. This is especially important if you are unfamiliar with the illness or what to expect. You can also find extremely valuable information on the Web sites of organizations that fight specific illnesses. The more you can anticipate what may be coming down the road, the better prepared all of you can be, physically, mentally, and emotionally.

Initial Guidelines for Hiring Professional Help: The Agency

We recommend the team take charge of researching, interviewing, hiring, troubleshooting, and overseeing all communications with the home-care agencies. They can start by asking for recommendations from others who have employed aides, from the hospital, or from the doctor handling your loved one's case. Plan to talk to several agencies, if you are lucky enough to have choices, and find out what they charge (negotiate if you can). Check with your friend's medical (or long-term care) insurance company *prior* to starting, as they may allow you to hire only from an approved agency. Verify that the agency is *Medicare Certified*, which means they will accept reimbursement from a third party. Also check to see they are licensed by the state and accredited by its professional association.

If the agency requires any contracts to be signed for hiring, have an attorney or someone knowledgeable in this area look them over beforehand. The person to sign them should be the one with your friend's power of attorney.

Interviewing the Health-Care Worker

Interview as many suitable candidates as possible. Ideally two team members should participate in the first interview, so afterward they can discuss their individual reactions to the candidate. We met our candidates in a bookstore café where we could sit off in a corner for some time, have a coffee, and talk. It seemed to work well.

When hiring a professional caregiver, it is vital to trust your intuition as well as your common sense. Just having the right certification may not be enough. Be very specific about what you need, and ask if that person can deliver. The agency may also have job descriptions about what aides are and are not required (or allowed) to do by law. Certain types of caregiving require different levels of training; an aide cannot do everything a registered nurse can. (If unsure, ask the hospital or physician what level of care your friend needs.)

Plan to tell the agency and the aide about your Share The Care group—what it is and how it works, and that the aide will be a most welcome addition. Make a list of questions to ask the aide at the interview, and give them a chance to ask you some as well. Some ideas:

- Do they have the level of skills your loved one's care will require? (Ask for photocopies or faxes of their credentials from the agency.)
- Do they have written recommendations? Read the letters and call the people who wrote them to ask some questions. It is the *only* way to find out how dependable someone really is.
- Check to see if they are currently licensed and registered with the state (State Department of Health, or Board of Regents, using name or Social Security Number).
- Have they cared for someone with   (your friend's specific disease) before?

- Have they cared for someone elderly who may be confused, or agitated (if applicable)?
- Do they seem flexible and patient?
- Do they have a sense of humor?
- Do they understand and speak English clearly?
- Are they in good health?
- Do they drive?
- Can they prepare simple meals for the person who is ill?
- Do they give you the impression that they really care about the work they do?
- Do they know how to operate lifts? Suction equipment? Feeding tubes? (What does your loved one require?)
- How long have they been employed by the agency?
- Will there be any restrictions on your loved one's end? No smoking is allowed in the house . . . is that a problem? There is a cat . . . are they allergic? There is a dog in the house . . . do they like dogs?

If, after your first meeting, you like the candidate, then schedule a meeting with your loved one and be observant. If your loved one is not well enough or cannot speak or is in any way unable to be part of the process, then it will be up to the team to make the best selection. If the care recipient can be involved the team should notice:

- How do they interact with your loved one?
- Are they gentle?
- Do they communicate directly with the person who is ill?
- Are they patient?
- How does your loved one respond to them?
- Ask the candidate if they have specific questions for you or the care recipient.

You Also Need Relief Workers

Assuming your loved one needs round-the-clock care, once you find the right person, you will *also* need to find a relief person or two. If you have interviewed lots of candidates perhaps there was a runner-up who would be a great relief person. Remember you need someone there on holidays (pay is usually double), weekends, and so forth. No one person can do this job without time off.

Living or Staying Overnight in the Home

If the person you hire is to be living in the home, plan to make some adjustments so they can have a room of their own. It should be next to or very close to the patient in case they are needed in the middle of the night. Devise a way for the person who is ill to call for them at night using a bell, buzzer, or intercom. Put a comfortable chair in your loved one's room so the aide can sit comfortably with them for long periods.

Briefing the Aide

Be friendly and establish rapport. Ask them what they would like to be called, Mary or Ms. Jones? Take them on a guided tour of what they need to know about the house and property. Introduce them to the entire family, neighbors, and the group members. Familiarize them with the Yellow Pages and any emergency procedures (which hospital emergency room should the patient be taken to, whom to call first, the directions to the home for EMS). Give them copies of everyone's contact numbers and the Telephone Tree. Show them how things work around the house. Remind them to ask if they are unsure about how to operate anything. Brief them about your loved one's likes or dislikes. Show them the Central Medical File containing Medical History, Medication Charts, Dosage Schedule, and Living Will. You might invite them to contribute to the Observation Journal, but realize they may prefer to create their own version. Then, let the aide do his or her job.

Your Group and the Aide

Make sure the Share The Care group members give the aide a warm welcome. Get things off to a good start. It's all about *teamwork*. Members should offer to help with the jobs that require more than one set of hands. Ask the aide to teach you something. The better everyone gets along, the better it is for the patient, who will surely detect any power plays going on. Any requests for the aide to do something should come from the captains. Remind the group that the aide is there specifically to care for the person who is ill, not to do other jobs around the house or help out other family members or children. Make it clear to the aide that if there are any problems or they need to work out an issue, they should contact one of the team members who hired them (give them both names and numbers) or communicate through the agency.

If Something Isn't Working, Get It Cleared Up Right Away

If within a couple of weeks of hiring an aide (nurse, companion, housekeeper), things don't seem to be working smoothly, have the hiring team member start by calmly discussing the issue with the employee to see if it can be easily resolved. Or if you prefer, communicate through the agency. Give the aide an opportunity to make adjustments to whatever is bothering you. For example: they seem to take and make an unusually large number of personal phone calls throughout the day, and this upsets the patient. Ask them to limit their calls to when the patient is napping. If the problem continues, let the agency know and ask them to start looking for a replacement right away. While this degree of friction, is rare, if it does occur it is best to make changes as soon as possible, before the patient becomes fearful or upset at the thought of having to get used to yet another person.

There are many wonderful, compassionate, hardworking men and women in the caring professions. The most valuable gift they can give is their loving care and companionship. When it is working well, there will be a beautiful bonding, and trust will occur between the patient and this most intimate caregiver.

A Special Bond Between Professional Caregiver and the Patient

During her final weeks at home, when she couldn't leave her bed, Susan had Laura, a truly special home health-care nurse who stayed with her even when she went into the hospice, and who was there when she died. The love, care, and tenderness with which she treated our dying friend was so great it was as if she had been sent from heaven in order to make the passage a little easier. Her presence allowed Susan's natural family and her caregiver family relief from the actual hands-on care during Susan's last weeks at home so that we could just "be there" to say our final good-byes.

When Caregiving at Home Is No Longer Possible

There are times when no matter how heroic the efforts of the group and nurse's aides might be, they can no longer keep up with the difficult and demanding kind of care a certain illness may require. It is important to realize when institutionalized care is needed. Though very painful to those who have given their all, it may be the only solution. Even if this occurs, your group can still make a difference by overseeing your friend's care from the outside. Here's a real-life example.

Going from Home Care to Institutionalized Care

The following words of advice are from Susan, a member of Nadine's Army of Angels. Nadine died in 2002 from complications due to amyotrophic lateral sclerosis (ALS). Nadine had no spouse and her immediate family lived far away. She was only forty-eight years old when she died. Her group worked hard to care for her when she could no longer do so for herself and to keep her at home for as long as possible. Armed with Share The Care and the help of the ALS Association, they were able to battle their own fears, frustrations, and grief to bring a little light into their friend's darkening life.

I can't emphasize enough how important it is to look ahead and be as prepared as possible for various contingencies. If it is a possibility that the seriously ill person is going to have to go to a nursing home eventually, start looking *now*. Many places will not take anyone under 60–65. Sometimes things happen very quickly and it is best to have a plan. Even someone who is being taken care of at home may end up in the hospital for a procedure and have to go to a nursing home before coming home again, so it's a good idea to know what is out there.

Because Nadine's condition became so bad she had to be institutionalized. We suggest maybe the most important thing to do for a seriously ill person who must be in a board-and-care or skilled nursing facility is to develop a good working relationship with as many of the staff members as possible. Even in the best facility, the staff are likely to be overworked and underpaid. They may bear the brunt of the frustration, anger, boredom, and fear of the person who is ill. They too, get burnt out, feel underappreciated and overwhelmed. Remember to thank workers who are kind and thoughtful. Regularly bringing treats (homemade cookies, pies, cake, etc.) in your friend's name can generate good will.

It was our experience that most of the staff at the nursing home where Nadine stayed were not familiar with ALS, the disease our friend had, and associated her speech difficulties and mood swings with diminished cognitive capacity. Since our friend had lost much of her capacity to speak by the time she was in a nursing home, we found it useful to help the staff get to know her by one-on-one conversations (we talked with the staff about Nadine—not just her disease but who *she* was).

We also created a laminated "bio" sheet, to help them see her as real person and not just another case. We printed, laminated, and hung by the bed lists of our friend's most common needs and questions. Since many of the staff did not speak or read English well, we made lists in both English and Spanish. The staff could then point to different items for a nod yes or no if they were having trouble understanding what she needed.

Caregiving Far from Home

Clinical Trials, Alternative Treatments, or Long Stays for Special Care

During their illnesses, both Susan and Cappy chose to try alternative treatments, which meant spending long periods away from home. The treatment Cappy decided to undertake in Houston required someone to be with her 24/7 for a couple of months to learn and monitor the equipment her treatment required. Normally, a family member would take on this role. Cappy was single, and none of her group could be away for such an extended period. So we searched through an agency for a suitable aide and found Christina. Though a registered nurse with very strong credentials in her native Zimbabwe, she was working as an aide until she could be certified in the United States. She possessed a very gentle nature. The minute she met Cappy you could tell they trusted each other. Christina proved to be wonderful. She was competent, observant, and totally dedicated to our friend, giving her the most loving care right to the very end.

Even though Cappy had Christina, she wanted and needed the companionship and leadership of someone she knew well. So Eileen, a veteran of Susan's Funny Family, became responsible for organizing the initial arrangements of the Houston Team, as they were dubbed. The friends who followed, heading for Texas for a week at a time, were mostly from other parts of the country. And they met with some big challenges when Cappy's condition slid into a rapid decline. While in Houston, her ability to communicate and walk diminished to zero and she needed a wheelchair full-time. She suffered other setbacks including emergency surgery, which literally saved her life. Had Cappy not desperately believed in this treatment, we would have brought her home much, much sooner. In the end, the treatment just didn't work for her.

An Undertaking Not to Be Taken Lightly

Caregiving at a distance is a serious challenge, yet sometimes it is the patient's only hope. It cannot be stressed enough that choosing alternative treatments or experimental trials requires the utmost in careful consideration, research, planning, and commitment by the group. Members who are part of the distant caregiving team need to be prepared emotionally for just about anything. We hope what Cappy's group learned can save others in a similar situation a lot of grief. Below, two members describe what it felt like to be "out there" on your own.

> It's just hard for people who aren't there to really know what goes on day to day. It can feel isolating being in a strange city, caring for a sick friend,

finding your way around, dealing with doctors you don't know who have unknown credentials. (K.M.)

It was as if we were on an island, away from everything and everyone familiar. (E.B)

Passing the Torch

One thing we brought with us from the first Funny Family experience far from home was the need to have a day to acclimate the new incoming helper before the one leaving actually makes their departure. This "changing of the guard" allowed routines to continue uninterrupted. The new person would be brought up to speed with a trip to the clinic, directions, and the personal input of the caregiver they were relieving. (How is the care recipient *really* doing emotionally? Are there any special signals from them if something is wrong?)* Pretending that it isn't hard doesn't fly. A truthful understanding of what to expect will leave the new person in a stronger position to cope.

This extra day made the transition for Cappy a little nicer as she enjoyed having both friends together for a day. It also gave the caregivers a little time to get to know each other, as they were usually from different parts of the country.

Anticipate, Research, and Plan Ahead with Airlines, Trains, and Buses

Whether it is alerting the airlines that you need bulkhead seats (the first row of seats in the cabin facing the wall), which are much roomier, or a courtesy wheelchair at both ends of the trip, do so well in advance of your flight and confirm the arrangements again the day before. *Confirming things is a good practice to get into.* You will be able to board early if your loved one requires special care such as a wheelchair or a walker. Generally, the airline personnel will go out of their way to make sure you are well taken care of. Make sure any medications and supplies required on the

---

* Reviewing entries in the Observation Journal (chapter 15) is also helpful.

trip are easily accessible. It would also be smart to carry a large bottle of water with you.

Plan for at least two people to travel with a patient who is in a wheelchair—one to tend to the patient's needs, the other to deal with tickets, luggage, transportation, security checks, and everything else that crops up.

If you are traveling by train or bus, call the carrier well in advance and find out how they might help make your trip easier. Traveling-with-disability information can be found on the Web site of the company you are traveling with, or give them a call and ask for customer service.

If it is at all possible, ship as much luggage and equipment as you can ahead to your destination rather than traveling with ten suitcases. In this age of multiple security checks at airports, it would be well worth the cost to not be burdened by looking for missing luggage or trying to fit everything into one car.

Free Air Transportation

Corporate Angels Network provides free air travel on corporate jets for cancer patients and bone-marrow donors and recipients, to and from treatment. There are some very specific restrictions, so check their Web site for details: http://www.corpangelnetwork.org. Also check Angel Flight NE at http://www.angelflightne.org, as they provide free air transportation for people with all kinds of illness or those who are accident victims.*

Build Extra Time into the Schedule

Traveling with someone who is ill or elderly also requires a good deal of extra time, so build it into your schedule. Avoid traveling at rush hour. Don't think you can whisk through the airport as you would under normal circumstances. Just because you are traveling with someone who is disabled in some way, don't assume things will move more easily for you, either. Quite the contrary, you may end up having a long wait for a courtesy

* See the Helpful Associations (Transportation/Housing) section at the back of the book for full contact information.

wheelchair to arrive. (Tip: When you have no control over what's happening, practice the mantra "I release").

Just getting into your seats will test your patience and that of your fellow travelers. When traveling, most people have a very low patience threshold. Be sure to thank others for their courtesy. You may find they will be especially helpful stowing your baggage or changing seats to accommodate your group. Whatever happens, though, try to keep your cool. It is crucial that the person you are caring for not feel pressured, as it could bring on an anxiety attack or breathing problems.

Hotels, Motels, and Apartments

Usually you can find good hotels, motels (with cooking facilities), or short-stay apartments near large clinics or hospitals because a steady stream of people come into town for treatment. Ask your contact at the hospital or clinic if they have a roster of recommendations. Often their sources will offer discounts for patients and their companions. Some health centers or clinics even provide free housing (ask if this is an option). See the Helpful Associations section (Transportation/Housing) at the back of the book to find addresses for the National Association of Hospital Hospitality Houses and the American Cancer Society's Hope Lodge Program. If your funds are limited and you are taking a child for treatment, check for a Ronald McDonald House in the area: http://www.rmhc.com.

If traveling with a wheelchair or walker, let the hotel/motel know ahead of time so they don't book you into a difficult-to-reach room at the far end of the building or up a flight of stairs.

Realize that it is a big strain to care for someone with physical problems in a hotel room. You may need to purchase, rent, or ship additional equipment to even make it possible, such as a bedside commode, a wheelchair, bath chair, rubber mats, and a handheld shower spray. Ask the clinic for the names of nearby medical supply stores that can deliver the draw sheets, rubber mattress cover, syringes, Ensure, colostomy bags, or whatever else you need directly to the hotel prior to your arrival. Note the telephone numbers and names of helpful salespeople.

Cars and Transportation

There were two other major reasons why Cappy needed someone besides Christina in Houston: Christina didn't have a driver's license, and Cappy suffered seizures that would manifest without warning. It would have been impossible to drive while this was occurring.

Do you know how you are going to get around a strange city or town? Don't expect cabs to be lined up at every corner. Outside of New York City, if one calls a cab it could take an hour or more before pickup. This is not a good option. Having a car is a necessity, so take this factor into consideration when figuring costs. Plan to locate a map of the city and become familiar with the lay of the land ahead of time.

If your loved one is in a wheelchair and cannot get in and out of it and the car without great difficulty, you may need an ambulette service. Ask the clinic, or try the hotel front desk or concierge for recommendations. Prearrange your transportation from the airport to the hotel and to and from the clinic and hotel. You may also want to plan some visits to a mall or park at some point for recreational purposes. Build in some sightseeing, entertainment, or fun time or else you will be very cranky.

The mayor's office in New York City offers a small paperback booklet, *Access in New York*, listing all of the transportation, sightseeing interests, restaurants, theaters, subway stations, and buses with accessibility for wheelchairs. Perhaps the mayor's office, chamber of commerce, or visitor's bureau in the city you will be visiting has a similar booklet, or can direct you to where you can find this extremely valuable information.

Meals and Shopping

Check to see if the hotel or motel has a restaurant or room service. Are there other nearby places to eat? (Be specific—you may have a Japanese sushi restaurant in mind and the front desk clerk may consider a fast-food place a prime option.) If you want to prepare some home-cooked meals once in a while to save on expenses, look for accommodations with cooking facilities. That way, you can whip up some pasta or a burger or stick to a special diet. It's a nice option to have, especially after a tiring day, when all any of you want to do is just relax and not struggle to go anywhere.

However, Margot saw a need for special items in their little kitchen:

I went out to the store and bought a blender for smoothies and other comfort foods and supplies for the kitchen. For a long stay like that it was easy, for just a little money, to set up housekeeping so it was homier.

Get directions from the front desk to the closest food and drugstore shopping facilities. Food shopping may just turn out to be one of the highlights of your day after hours of sitting around a clinic waiting to see a doctor or have tests.

Laundry and Dry Cleaning

Does the hotel have a laundry service? Can you afford to pay for these services or are you on a tight budget? If cost is a consideration, find a local laundry/dry cleaner or laundromat if the motel doesn't have a laundry room. Pack clothes that can be thrown in the washer and dryer, and look good without ironing and you will be ahead of the game. Plan to make time to handle this chore. (Tip: Bring several rolls of quarters.)

In general, pack clothes for your loved one that are very comfortable, easy to get into, and require little care. Choose three or four basic colors or prints you can mix and match easily. Plan to dress your loved one in layers and bring along a sweater or shawl they can easily put on or drape as a lap robe over their legs. Even in the heat of summer you could arrive at the clinic and find that the air-conditioning feels like Antarctica. Older people and those who are ill don't always have good circulation and may feel cold even if you are sweltering. (Tip: Don't forget the umbrella.)

Entertainment on the Road

Ship or come armed with a variety of entertainment for everyone. There is nothing worse than sitting around a hotel room on a dreary, rainy day when there's not a thing worth watching on television. Bring a laptop computer (more about this necessity later), games, cards, puzzles (crossword and jigsaw), magazines, toys (if you have a child), writing paper, watercolors, colored pencils, and music. A camera would be great if you want to record this trip.

Do you love to write? Bring a journal. Learn a new language on tapes. Catch up on the novels you have never had time to read. Or, if you must, keep up with some office work or study for that real estate class you are taking.

Another rainy day suggestion is a "Spa Day." Play some relaxing classical or New Age tapes. Purchase some fragrant shampoo, bath gel, shaving creams, lotions, and a face mask. Spray the room with lavender or orange fragrance with your mist bottle.* Give your loved one a facial and a refreshing mask, then have them rest a bit with a cup of peppermint tea while you partake of some of this pampering yourself. Help them with a bath or shower, wash their hair, put on a fluffy robe and blow-dry their hair. Try some new hairstyles, or give them a shave and/or a manicure and pedicure. Then finish off with a foot rub or neck rub. Treat yourselves to room service or make a nice light dinner. You ought to sleep well after this high-intensity pampering. (Tip: Put a few drops of lavender oil on your pillowcase to be sure.)

CD players are great, but usually only the person with the headset gets to enjoy the CDs. Judy went out and purchased an inexpensive CD player so everyone in the room could enjoy the music. She also thought it would be helpful to play tapes for Cappy's speech therapy out loud. Singing was part of the therapy drill, and Cappy's little group ended up doing a "sing-along" with her every day, which made it seem more like fun.

There are some terrific portable DVD players available these days. If you have one, bring movies, games, or other entertainment to watch. Find a local video/DVD rental store if you need a better selection. Hint to the folks back home that sending new DVDs would be an ideal gift.

---

* See "Make Use of Aromatherapy," page 225.

Personalize Your Hotel Room

Ask for a nonsmoking room, for starters. The last thing you want is a room that has the traces of stale smoke for a long stay. Move the furniture around so it works for *you*. (Or ask to have it moved.) Does the bed need to be against the wall so your loved one doesn't roll out? Cover up the ugly painting with a pretty scarf. Tape up (with removable tape) an inexpensive or pretty poster. On occasion, get flowers to cheer up the room. Keep cards, photos, and postcards from well-wishers stuck in the rim of the mirror. Or purchase an inexpensive corkboard to display items or pin up numbers. Create a special area only for medications and things needed for treatment. Keep the room neat and smelling nice.

Communicating with the Group Back Home

Bring a laptop computer—you're going to need it. Plan to keep it with the patient for the entire stay and have it pre-programmed with all the needed group e-mail addresses. That way, no one has to bring his or her own laptop unless they choose to do so. E-mail is the most efficient and cost-effective way to stay in touch with the rest of your group, especially if you're in a different time zone. That way, help for the caregiver (practical and emotional) is only a mouse click away.

Anne, who is relatively new to computers, had a very valuable piece of advice on this subject:

> Prior to leaving home, have someone write up in very simple language how to start up and shut down the computer, how to send and receive e-mail, and how to get on the Internet. Not everyone is computer literate and able to figure out how to do even simple tasks without detailed instructions.

Those of us back in New York waited for the almost daily updates on how Cappy was doing emotionally and physically. Her Houston companions had the burden of reporting on their shoulders, and it wasn't always easy to paint the true picture. Some wise advice from Kathy:

The main group wants accurate information. The caretaker at a distance should give an accurate account of the situation, without sugarcoating it or trying to put a happy, perky spin on it. There's room for humor, of course, but tell it like it is, whatever it is. Also, if something was needed by the Houston Team, such as research, airline reservations, or special books and CDs that Cappy wanted from home, they could request that a New York team handle it.

It is very healing to know others are thinking of you and sending prayers, love, and good wishes. The group can keep these flowing by sending cards, letters, e-mails, flowers, or small gifts. Having some mail or messages waiting for you at the hotel can really brighten your day. Try to call occasionally so they can hear the sound of your voice, but don't overdo it.

You can also use a free Web site or a blog to communicate to the group about your friend's condition. This should be set up in advance of leaving home, by someone who is good at computer technology and who can provide clear written instructions for those who will be in charge of doing updates.

Local Contact Information, Addresses, Directions

Early on, Cappy's cousin Patty started a logbook that turned out to be a godsend for all who followed. The logbook and Yellow Pages went everywhere they did, so calls could be made at will on the cell phone. Plan to bring a blank notebook with you rather than wait to purchase one when you arrive. You could miss recording some really good information early on. Patty recalled:

> I started a notebook that I thought was very valuable. In it there were important phone numbers for Houston: clinic, pharmacy, doctors, pages of directions to important places such as food stores, "things to do" in Houston, and schedules. I left the notebook for the next person to use and add to.

If someone in your group has friends or family in the city you will be visiting, ask them for their contact information. Contact these people ahead of time to tell them they might get a call from a group member. These contacts could be extremely helpful for recommendations of all kinds from great restaurants to an emergency dentist.

Keep Important Papers, Bills, and Expenses Organized

Try your best to keep track of expenses or at the very least, keep receipts and records organized. Bring manila envelopes and mark them Hotel, Food, Medical Expenses, Miscellaneous, and so forth. Bring envelopes, stamps, lined yellow paper, stickies, scissors, paper clips, tape, and some manila folders or plastic envelopes with closures to keep important medical information. That way dropping papers in the mail to the person back home in charge of medical claims is a breeze.

Emergency Situations Far from Home

Medical emergencies are bad enough, but dealing with them in another city can really be frightening. One thing you can do to prepare for this possibility is to get some physician and hospital references ahead of time. Eileen offers some excellent advice about getting this kind of critical up-front research before leaving home:

> Find out in advance from the treatment facility exactly what would happen in a medical emergency and what doctors would be handling such an emergency. (The daily clinic doctor? An outside physician? A doctor assigned at the hospital emergency room?) In our case, the surgeon who had inserted Cappy's catheter had privileges at a local hospital, so she was admitted there as his patient. He happened to be a general surgeon and, when she needed emergency surgery, he did happen to do a very good job. Thank God. But other specialists had to be called in for other problems. . . . people we didn't know, who were not familiar with the clinic protocol (or not sympathetic to it). And the fact that the surgeon was Cappy's primary physician while she was in the hospital was not great. Again we had the situation where the surgeon was monitoring her recent surgery but perhaps was not the best person to be evaluating her *overall*

condition. A little research in this area would be wise so that you know how the facility handles such problems, and you can perhaps back yourself up with some reliable resources. Remember, if you are experimenting with an alternative treatment, not every hospital is going to welcome you.

Paying All the Expenses

Cappy was fortunate to be able to cover the expenses for her companion and Christina. Most of the weekly companions paid for their own transportation, but if someone couldn't afford the fare, Cappy was able to have one of us arrange for her airline miles to be transferred and a ticket issued in their name.

If someone in your group cannot afford the expense of airfare or hotel and the person who is ill cannot cover their expenses, consider these options: The group members could chip in some cash and/or donate their miles to that person. If there is some lead time, the group could do some kind of fund-raising (tag sale or cake sales) to pay for these worthwhile expenses. Use your imagination. Keep in mind that this person is not going on some exotic vacation but on a very challenging mission.

CHAPTER SEVENTEEN

Making the Home Safe and Comfortable

Hazards in the Home

Over time, our group found that we had to make many safety adjustments to Susan's New York apartment. These included getting rid of some elegant but dangerous throw rugs, having wires removed, rearranging some closets, and adding grab bars to the shower and bath. We probably should have moved a little faster to do these things, but we didn't realize the need for them right away.

We encourage your group to check out what might be a hazard in your friend's home now rather than waiting for an accident to happen. If your friend is recovering from a serious accident or surgery you may not have the luxury of waiting and will need to make adjustments immediately. Though many of our suggestions are not new or unusual, we feel it is important to remind you of the need for them.

What to Look For

Falls are one of the leading causes of accidental deaths, especially among the elderly. A fall can be a serious setback for someone already recovering from an injury. People who are unsteady on their feet due to illness are also at high risk for falling.

After one of her operations, Susan's arm was in a sling for a very long period of time. This made taking a shower extremely difficult and scary for her. Then one member suggested having grab bars installed at different levels (shower and bath) and adding a rubber bath mat to prevent slipping. Although she resisted at first, Susan later told us that the bars really made her feel more secure and she wished she'd had them put in sooner.

A Word of Caution Before You Start

If the person who is ill has a spouse or companion or lives with family members, the caregiver group must be very sensitive about suggesting changes within the home. The family is probably so preoccupied with their loved one's illness that doing a safety check of their surroundings is the last thing on their mind. This might be especially true if the person whose safety you are concerned about has suddenly been left physically impaired. Try to find at least two people within the group who are close to the family to take on this assignment.

Guidelines for Members Doing a House Safety Check

Talking to the Family

One of you, the one closest to the family, can suggest doing a house check with a family member or offer to do it yourselves and discuss it with them afterward.

- Tell them the group can find people to make repairs or buy needed equipment.
- Assure them the caregivers are there to help them, too.
- Don't pressure them; give them time to think it over.

Talking to the Patient

If patients have no live-in family, and especially if they are not in an advanced state of illness, they will probably resent any attempt the group makes to try to reorganize their home—and they may even tell you to mind your own business. They will be fearful of making changes and letting others take over, and will fight to stay as independent as possible, even though you can see certain dangers in their home.

In gentle, diplomatic ways, make suggestions periodically about repairs or improvements. "Maybe we should ask Bill to come over on Saturday and get these wires from the TV out of this doorway. . . . Someone could trip and fall." Or "Don't you think you should get a phone for your bedside? There is a sale down at the shopping center and I could pick one up for you tomorrow. That way you could call one of us if you needed anything." (If you purchase a new phone, get one that can be programmed with emergency numbers.)

Doing the House Check

Here are some suggestions of what to look for (room by room) in your friend's home or apartment. These are followed by charts (on pages 218 and 219) you can use as you do the check and note where repairs or purchases will be needed. The charts can also be used as reminders of whom you need to find for the repairs and to keep track of the jobs until they are completed.

THE OUTSIDE ENTRANCE

If your friend lives in an apartment building you may have to consult with the superintendent or co-op board in order to get certain things repaired, such as a broken hall light.

- Does the elevator work?
- Is there good security?
- Is there an automatic garage door opener?
- Is the mailbox close to the door? Can it be moved or a mail slot installed?
- Are there rails for the stairs? Can these be added?
- Do you need wheelchair access?*

* See chapter 15, "Finding Your Way Through the Medical Maze," for a discussion of special medical equipment.

THE INSIDE ENTRANCE

- If there are stairs, are they well lit on top and bottom? If there are rugs on the stairway, are they properly attached to the stairs?
- Keep clutter off the stairs—toys, shoes, etc.
- If the person has trouble seeing or is elderly, perhaps a colored strip can be added to the top stair and bottom stair so the different levels can be distinguished.
- If someone sleeping upstairs could be confused in the middle of the night, consider the use of a gate at the top of the stairs. If a stairway is truly proving to be a serious obstacle, suggest that the patient consider relocating the bedroom to the ground floor, if space permits (see the section on the bedroom, below).

THE LIVING ROOM

- Repair or get rid of all unstable furniture such as rickety chairs or tables, wobbly bookcases, uncomfortable seating. Nothing is worth keeping if it can cause injury.
- Do the TV and DVD player have remote controls so your friend doesn't have to keep getting up and down to turn them on and off?
- Rearrange furniture for comfort and convenience.

THE BATHROOM

- The bath and shower can be very dangerous places if the hot and cold faucets don't work properly. A sudden jolt of scalding water can cause a bad burn or startle someone into a fall.
- Intalling grab bars for the shower and bath is very important. They help the person feel more secure.
- A grab bar may also be necessary near the toilet. Find out if this would be a help.
- Get rubber mats for the inside of the bathtub.
- Does the person need a shower bench? Maybe he can't stand for long periods

of time. A bench can make showering easier. Also, if the patient needs help showering, a handheld attachment can be of great use.

- Are soap, shampoo, and so on, accessible? How about adding a shower shelf or caddy? The person should not have to bend down in the shower to pick things up off the floor.

- Is a higher toilet seat needed? This item can be purchased and attached easily.

THE KITCHEN

- The items that are used every day, such as the toaster and coffeemaker, should be easily accessible.

- Does the person have difficulty opening things? Nothing can be more frustrating even if you are healthy. Get an electric opener or special jar openers (made for people with arthritis or the elderly).

THE BEDROOM

- How is the bedside lighting? Can your friend see what he or she is doing while in bed? This will be especially important with medications.

- Is there a phone by the bed? If not, get one.

- Is there a clock?

- Is there room for the patient's medications? Susan's night table was initially so crowded that there was no place for even a glass of water. Eventually, we got rid of the clutter.

- Are there night lights leading to the bathroom? This is another essential item that costs almost nothing and is so simple to install.

- Help rearrange closets so the patient can get to the clothes and items needed on a daily basis.

- Does the patient need any special pillows or textured mattress covers for extra support and for extra comfort? See if the doctor has any special recommendations.

- Last, but most important, should the patient relocate the bedroom to a different floor? A successful example of such a move was when Sheila's mom started having difficulty climbing the stairs of her home every night. Sheila suggested she move to a spare room downstairs. Granted, it was smaller and not as nice, but it had an adjoining bathroom so her mom wouldn't have to walk down a long hallway in the middle of the night. The furniture was moved down and the room decorated to look as close to upstairs as possible. And her mom came to really like it because it was convenient, comfortable, and she didn't have to struggle with the stairs every morning and night.

MAKING THE PATIENT COMFORTABLE

- Is there comfortable seating? Can the patient stand up and sit down easily? Do his or her legs need to be elevated? Does the patient have back problems and need extra support? Check into getting a reclining chair made especially for people who have particular needs.
- Is there a good reading lamp? What about a desk, or a portable desk that fits across a chair or bed?
- Is there a place for the phone (including all numbers) close at hand? What about the pillbox, water, timer, books, magazines, and TV and DVD controls?
- Is a bell, buzzer, or intercom needed to signal someone in another part of the house?

(See chapter 15 for more specific information on where to find medical equipment, special furniture, and helpful gadgets.)

HOME SAFETY CHART

This form can be downloaded from the Web site.

Date: _____

SHARE THE CARE

(page 1)

CHECK THE FOLLOWING:	OUTSIDE ENTRANCE	INSIDE ENTRANCE	LIVING ROOM	BATHROOM	KITCHEN	BEDROOM
Lighting • Overhead lights • Hallways • Stairs	☐ Good ☐ Repairs needed ☐ Equipment needed notes:	☐ Good ☐ Repairs needed ☐ Equipment needed notes:	☐ Good ☐ Repairs needed ☐ Equipment needed notes:	☐ Good ☐ Repairs needed ☐ Equipment needed notes:	☐ Good ☐ Repairs needed ☐ Equipment needed notes:	☐ Good ☐ Repairs needed ☐ Equipment needed notes:
Wires • TV • DVD • Cable • Lamps • Fans • Fax	☐ Good ☐ Repairs needed ☐ Equipment needed notes:	☐ Good ☐ Repairs needed ☐ Equipment needed notes:	☐ Good ☐ Repairs needed ☐ Equipment needed notes:	☐ Good ☐ Repairs needed ☐ Equipment needed notes:	☐ Good ☐ Repairs needed ☐ Equipment needed notes:	☐ Good ☐ Repairs needed ☐ Equipment needed notes:
Smoke Alarm • Are the batteries working? • Does one need to be installed? Where?	☐ Good ☐ Repairs needed ☐ Equipment needed notes:	☐ Good ☐ Repairs needed ☐ Equipment needed notes:	☐ Good ☐ Repairs needed ☐ Equipment needed notes:	☐ Good ☐ Repairs needed ☐ Equipment needed notes:	☐ Good ☐ Repairs needed ☐ Equipment needed notes:	☐ Good ☐ Repairs needed ☐ Equipment needed notes:
Unstable Furniture • Wobbly furniture • Sharp edges on tables	☐ Good ☐ Repairs needed ☐ Equipment needed notes:	☐ Good ☐ Repairs needed ☐ Equipment needed notes:	☐ Good ☐ Repairs needed ☐ Equipment needed notes:	☐ Good ☐ Repairs needed ☐ Equipment needed notes:	☐ Good ☐ Repairs needed ☐ Equipment needed notes:	☐ Good ☐ Repairs needed ☐ Equipment needed notes:

HOME SAFETY CHART

This form can be downloaded from the Web site.

SHARE THE CARE

Date: _____ (page 2)

CHECK THE FOLLOWING:	OUTSIDE ENTRANCE	INSIDE ENTRANCE	LIVING ROOM	BATHROOM	KITCHEN	BEDROOM
Rugs • Are they secured to the floor? • Remove throw rugs	☐ Good ☐ Repairs needed ☐ Equipment needed notes:	☐ Good ☐ Repairs needed ☐ Equipment needed notes:	☐ Good ☐ Repairs needed ☐ Equipment needed notes:	☐ Good ☐ Repairs needed ☐ Equipment needed notes:	☐ Good ☐ Repairs needed ☐ Equipment needed notes:	☐ Good ☐ Repairs needed ☐ Equipment needed notes:
Stairs • Are rugs secured to the stairs? • Do you need a gate?	☐ Good ☐ Repairs needed ☐ Equipment needed notes:	☐ Good ☐ Repairs needed ☐ Equipment needed notes:	☐ Good ☐ Repairs needed ☐ Equipment needed notes:	☐ Good ☐ Repairs needed ☐ Equipment needed notes:	☐ Good ☐ Repairs needed ☐ Equipment needed notes:	☐ Good ☐ Repairs needed ☐ Equipment needed notes:
Special Equipment • Grab Bars • Shower chair • Toilet seat	☐ Good ☐ Repairs needed ☐ Equipment needed notes:	☐ Good ☐ Repairs needed ☐ Equipment needed notes:	☐ Good ☐ Repairs needed ☐ Equipment needed notes:	☐ Good ☐ Repairs needed ☐ Equipment needed notes:	☐ Good ☐ Repairs needed ☐ Equipment needed notes:	☐ Good ☐ Repairs needed ☐ Equipment needed notes:
General Repairs Needed • Air conditioner • Heating • Windows • Doors • Fans • Washer/dryer • Dishwasher	☐ Good ☐ Repairs needed ☐ Equipment needed notes:	☐ Good ☐ Repairs needed ☐ Equipment needed notes:	☐ Good ☐ Repairs needed ☐ Equipment needed notes:	☐ Good ☐ Repairs needed ☐ Equipment needed notes:	☐ Good ☐ Repairs needed ☐ Equipment needed notes:	☐ Good ☐ Repairs needed ☐ Equipment needed notes:

CHAPTER EIGHTEEN

Beyond Safety and Comfort

Making Life More Pleasant

While you are getting things in place in terms of safety and comfort, try to also consider the home from yet another perspective—the senses. Looking at the home in this way can be especially beneficial for someone confined to bed all day staring at the same walls day in and day out. You, as caregivers, probably already have your hands full, so these tips may not appear at the top of your to-do list, but they do play a big part in how your loved one feels on a day-to-day basis.

What Do They Look At All Day?

Try this test when your loved one is in another room or out of the house. Put yourself in their bed or wheelchair for a couple of minutes and check out what they look at all day long. It can be a very enlightening exercise. Believe it or not, someone's surroundings can become their "view of life," which in turn affects their outlook and ability to want to get better. If the room is dreary, dark, dirty, messy, and cluttered, pay attention as your loved one may already be showing signs of depression and hopelessness. Here's what can be done to raise their spirits pretty easily.

Start by asking how they feel about their bedroom. See if they'd like to have their room rearranged or to move the position of their bed for a change. Perhaps they want to move to another room entirely, or try spending time in another part of the house, at least during the day. Walk around with them, if possible, and consider the possibilities.

- Is there another room with more pleasant views of nature or some activity that would provide some positive stimulation? Or conversely, do they need to be in a more peaceful and quiet setting?
- Who says you can't transform the dining room, living room, or den into a bedroom? Maybe they feel isolated and forgotten on the second floor, so just by moving to the first floor the patient feels more connected to the family, and this will save the caregivers the tedious job of climbing stairs all day.
- Make sure the patient can see who is coming through the door of their re-arranged bedroom or new bedroom. You never want to startle them or have them strain to see who has come into their room. If it's not possible to change the bed position, then hang a mirror so they can see the door from their vantage point in bed.
- Note that a lot of mirrors in a home can be disconcerting to someone who is confused or has very bad vision. If illness has taken a toll on someone's appearance, they may prefer *not* to see their image constantly reflected everywhere they go in the house. Put some of these mirrors away.
- If their room is particularly dark, you may want to consider purchasing a sun box* that floods a room with light and makes it feel like a sunny day. These lighting fixture are commonly used by people who become depressed during the winter months (seasonal affective disorder, or SAD), when the sun is less visible.

If it is a matter of getting the patient out of the bedroom for the day, figure out what they'd like to be doing right then. Remember it may change day to day. If they are into cable TV or watching movies on DVDs set them up in the family room or the den—wherever the biggest TV screen is located. If the weather is nice and they are lucky enough to have a patio, porch, terrace, or little garden, encourage them to sit outside and enjoy some fresh air and sunshine.

* See Helpful Associations (Equipment) at the back of the book for the Sunbox Web site.

The Downside of Technology

We live in an incredible world of technology filled with computers, printers, cell phones, TVs, DVDs, and microwaves. As wonderful as all these machines can be, they produce electromagnetic fields that have a physical impact on us. Imagine how much more draining these invisible waves are for someone who is fighting for their very life. Give a patient every chance possible to gain strength and rest while in bed and not be zapped of their energy. Be aware of *where* you place their bed and *what* surrounds them. Move large pieces of equipment (TVs, computers) away from the bed and into another room if possible. Skip the electric blankets and opt for down feather covers. Do not have twelve electrical cords plugged into the outlet right next to the head of their bed. Do not have the head of any bed on the same wall as the electrical outlet box for the entire house. (Can you imagine how much electricity is pouring through that wall?) Don't put the head of the bed against the wall where there is a huge refrigerator, freezer, or a lot of office equipment plugged into the other side of the same wall. Keep the head of the bed off the same wall as the toilet or bathtub as well.

Get Rid of the Mess and Clutter

Get rid of any mess or clutter in the bedroom, in fact, in *all* the rooms. Nothing drains one's energy and makes a person feel "stuck and confused" so quickly as looking at piles of clothes and clutter. Stacks of newspapers or magazines or boxes of "junk" just weigh down a room and are dust collectors. Store nothing under the bed. Leave no trays of half-eaten food or filled-up wastebaskets sitting around. Everyone in the house will benefit once the clutter has been cleared and the place gets a really good cleaning. You'll notice instantly that things seem brighter, lighter, and your loved one will respond positively to how fresh the house looks and feels.

Get rid of everything in the bedroom that your loved one doesn't really like, and surround them with the things they love, use, have a sentimental attachment to, or find beautiful. That could mean anything from a beautiful antique to their grandson's rendering of a fish. Beauty, in this case, is always in the eye of the person who is ill. This point was driven home to me when I asked a seriously ill friend why she had an illustration of a fierce samurai warrior hanging in her bathroom—he was so angry looking. Her response just blew me away: "In the morning when I have my bath, I look at his face and he gives me the strength to go on. I can see the warrior in myself."

If your loved one has the strength to participate in clearing the clutter, it could be an excellent thing for them to do. Janet, a former free-floater in Susan's group, was in the beginning stages of ALS when she decided clearing clutter from her tiny apartment was a great suggestion. She took control of doing it, and this act turned out to be a major cathartic experience as well as an empowering one. Janet meticulously went through all of her personal papers and belongings and filed, threw away, or gave away whatever she felt she no longer needed. It made her incredibly happy to have accomplished her goal.

A Little Extra Effort

Try to keep fresh flowers around (but don't keep them once they start to wilt). They are one of Mother Nature's most nurturing gifts. If the care recipient's favorite flowers are out of season or you can't afford new ones every week, invest in a pretty arrangement of their favorite flowers in silk—but skip the plastic kind. A colorful bowl of oranges or mixed fruit might be just the thing to perk up someone's appetite if they haven't been eating. Even the way you serve their meals can have an impact. Use those colorful place mats, napkins, and the pretty china. What are you saving them for anyway? Let them enjoy the "good stuff." Make them feel special.

The Power of Color

For centuries color has been used for healing. In fact, just painting a room a new color can be one of the most inexpensive ways to instantly cheer someone up. Consider painting just one or two walls (the ones they look at) with a color that resonates with the patient. Remember you can always paint over it. Or redecorate with their favorite colors: new curtains, a bedspread, or throw pillows for the bed or couch in soft greens and lavenders.

Hang a grouping of paintings or photographs in similar hues. Pretty new sheets can immediately create a sense of well-being. If you have an interior designer or artist in your group, have them make suggestions, but be sure you work with colors that the patient really likes. It makes sense to keep bedroom colors soft, though not necessarily pale, and to use small accents of brighter colors. Bright colors sometimes can make sleeping or resting difficult. Avoid bright reds, oranges, and bright yellows in the bedroom, especially for a person who is seriously ill.

Getting Dressed

Have you ever noticed when you wear certain colors you feel more powerful, pretty, or confident? So use color to the patient's advantage: If they need a little boost of energy, wearing strong colors could be the ticket—vibrant pinks, periwinkle blues, or daffodil yellow. If the person is generally nervous or irritable, stick with wardrobe colors in cooler, more neutral shades—pale or denim blues, soft celery greens, or heather gray—that are calming to the spirit.

In terms of the elderly, if you need to shop for their clothes, keep your choices true to who they are. Don't make the mistake of trying to dress someone who has always been conservative and tailored in things that are fussy, bright, or patterned with bold flowers. Stick to what they always liked—subtle checks, or simple prints. Keep them in colors they like and that look good on them. Make sure items are easy to pull on, zip, or snap, or have big buttons. Older people and those who are seriously ill don't have the strength or agility to struggle with getting something on or off. Make it easy so getting dressed isn't some form of torture.

When someone reaches a point in their illness where they only wear very basic, easy-to-pull-on clothes or hospital-type gowns, do them a favor and move their other things to the back of the closet or into another room so they don't have to be reminded of what they can't fit into or wear anymore.

If your friend has started chemotherapy and is losing hair, she may be understandably bummed out. She may or may not go for the idea of a wig, as many patients today embrace their baldness while undergoing treatment. It will depend on the individual. You might be able to lift her spirits by giving her a hat party. Ask the group and other friends to come up with their best finds: scarves, turbans, floppy hats, berets, beanies, headbands, hats with horns, hats with sequins, hats with flowers, gold hats, denim hats—the choices are endless. Who knows, maybe you can also create hats that *all* the members can wear. Envision the group of you in bright red baseball caps emblazed with the name "Trina's Tribe."

Make Use of Aromatherapy

A patient's room may sometimes have an unpleasant odor, so air it out whenever possible, especially on a warm, sunny day. We suggest rather than spraying the room with harsh chemical air fresheners, you try a little aromatherapy. For centuries, people have believed essential oils have positive benefits for our mind, body, and emotions. Fill a small spray mist bottle with water and add 15–20 drops of an aromatherapy essential oil. Just make sure you purchase real therapeutic essential oils (not chemical fragrances); otherwise there can be no positive effect.

Cappy and Sheila spent many years developing new fragrances, and part of the job meant learning about aromatherapy. It was natural to incorporate this practice into the daily routine during Cappy's illness. The following are general aromatherapy guidelines for getting started. The oils are sold in small brown or blue bottles, usually in health food stores. The individual price may vary depending on the choice of oil. Below are some suggestions for the basic ones to start. The best two to start with are lavender and orange.

- *Lavender* is excellent for use at bedtime as it aids relaxation and soothes the nerves, making it possible to sleep more easily. Put a few drops of lavender on a tissue; inhaling the scent can instantly calm someone who is agitated or nervous. It's a good oil to take with you in the car or to the doctor, and especially while traveling by air.
- *Orange or lemon* can be uplifting, refreshing, and enlivening. Either choice is good for clearing the air of anger, worry, or anxiety. Just spray some around if

there have been harsh words or tears in the room. The negativity will dissipate and everyone's demeanor will be more calm.

- *Eucalyptus* has a very balancing effect, especially if someone is feeling irrational or moody. It's also good for opening the breathing passages, and a few drops in a bath—but just a few—relaxes muscles.
- *Rose* is very good to balance and purify the air. If someone is fond of roses, this is a real winner. Rose embodies a heart-warming and calming fragrance.

Others scents to consider: *geranium, neroli, rosewood,* and *peppermint.*

Never apply essential oils directly on the skin. They need to be mixed with a carrier oil (such as apricot oil or almond oil) before use as massage oil. Always ask about oils, other than those mentioned here, as some should not used by pregnant women or should be used infrequently. Check the essential oil chart at the counter or ask someone at the store who is familiar with the line. There are many good books, articles, and Web sites where you can learn more about aromatherapy.*

Another option that we found very pleasing was Florida Water.† We put it straight into a mist bottle and sprayed it around the house daily, several times a day. It's an old-fashioned Victorian cologne with a subtle orangey fragrance. In New York it can be purchased in drugstores in Chinatown or Spanish bodegas and is inexpensive though sometimes difficult to find. Florida Water is used full-strength not only as a room spray but also as an aftershave, skin freshener, and palliative for insect bites.

The Noise Factor

What sounds can be heard from your friend's bedroom? Traffic noise, screaming children at a nearby school playground, loud neighbors, or sounds of construction? (Any of these could be reason to move a bedroom.) Besides keeping the windows closed, what can you do about it? If a

---

* See Special Interest Books on page 324.

† One online source for Murray & Lanman's Florida Water cologne is Montreal's Cordially Yours (prices are given in U.S. dollars): http://www.cordiallyyours.net/african_american asian_caribbean_shopping/item3046.htm.

lot of street noise in the evening interferes with the patient's sleep, try a sound machine programmed with soothing nature sounds: the ocean, rain, birds, wind or white noise.

If the person who is ill thrives on music, get them a decent CD player (with a good, comfortable headset) to override the endless noise from outside. CDs are a great gift idea for people far away looking for something to send as a gift. Taped personal messages instead of a letter are another way for their loved one to enjoy personal news and stories.

Activities That Keep Them Involved in Life

If your loved one is fortunate they will have a skill or hobby that fills their day and sometimes becomes the way they *keep living*. Make their work accessible: a special table with the model airplane materials neatly organized; the watercolor paper, brushes, and paint; or a laptop computer with printer and paper so they can write their short stories or surf the Web. Encourage them if they want to undertake writing up family stories or a special adventure in their life. Perhaps they would have an interest in creating a family album out of all the old pictures stored in the attic. Help out in every way possible to satisfy their need to feel productive or creative. If they can't indulge in an old pastime, encourage them to try something new that they might be able to handle.

Using the Internet for Entertainment and Learning

Some activities or interests can be enhanced by the vast number of resources that are available on the Internet. These suggestions were contributed by Steve from Cappy's Brain Trust.

The Internet can be a huge boon to a shut-in. Virtually anything you can buy, rent, eat, wear, use, borrow, sell, or play with can be ordered up and delivered right to your house.

- Does your friend love movies? Go to http://www.netflix.com, a movie-by-mail service. Order as many films as you want, watch them, and then send them back in the prepaid self-mailers Netflix provides.

- Don't forget the simple gift of upgrading someone's cable service. Cappy used to love the movies—and as she got less mobile, we upgraded her cable so she could get all the premium movie channels. For an extra $30 a month, she could enjoy many of the films she'd missed.

- Does your friend love books but have trouble reading? Books on tape and CD are available to rent or buy. Try http://www.audible.com and http://www.booksontape.com; both offer CD-Rom or audiotape books for rental or purchase by mail.

- Trouble writing? Speech recognition software is becoming much more reliable. A group member can set up the computer so the person can just put on a headset or speak into the microphone and the computer will automatically type out e-mail, pick the correct address, and send and receive your e-mail.

- Both Windows and Mac software have built-in options for special needs. Again, you should ask a computer-savvy member or friend to stop by and help set up your (patient's) computer to match their needs: larger icons, special fonts, voice recognition software, ergonomic keyboard, and so on. And if it's not available already on the computer, chances are you can find it with a simple Internet search.

CHAPTER NINETEEN

When Groups Help Out at Home

When Everyone Needs Easy Access

At some point in your friend's illness he or she may not be able to get up to open the front door for group members all day without a lot of stress and strain. How you choose to resolve the issue of access will depend a lot on the kind of community you live in and the level of security everyone feels is important. Here are two drastically different examples.

The Open Door Policy— Santa Fe, New Mexico

Rick lived with his wife, Mary, in Santa Fe. He suffered from kidney cancer and during the course of his illness he traveled out of state to undergo two operations to remove a tumor from his spine. Neither surgery proved successful, and due to an enormous blood loss he was rendered blind as well. Back home Camille, the coordinator, and his group of thirty-three men and women organized to become a Share The Care group. To make their visits less interruptive, the front door was always left unlocked (during the day) and posted with a sign that said Please Come In, so the group, family, and other friends could come and go at will. A Welcome Center was set up just inside the front door with a bulletin board and a large erasable calendar. It brought everyone up-to-date on Rick's condition daily so group members would know what to expect or how quiet to be when they went to his room. The group could also leave messages for each other, which provided a close sense of community. People experienced it as a haven. Even if the Open Door part of this idea is not a possibility, making a Welcome Center for your group is a relatively simple matter.

Safety First—New York City

Susan's group was located in Manhattan, known for having apartments with multiple locks, doormen, and security devices. Susan was unable to get around easily, and while she was happy with our comings and goings it was sometimes annoying and difficult for her to get up to answer the door. So she agreed that the group should have keys to the building's front door as well as keys to her apartment. When her illness left her bedridden, this turned out to be a real blessing.

If the patient agrees that this is a good idea, the captain can assign the job of having the keys made. They should be labeled and distributed to the group. Members should keep their keys with them at all times so they can always have access.

As a courtesy to Susan, the members always called to tell her we were on our way up to her apartment so she wouldn't be frightened or startled at hearing a key in her front door. A neighbor who was a member had keys to her mailbox and collected the mail for her daily.

If the person has a car, keep the car keys in one central place in case a member needs to drive the car to a doctor's appointment, run an errand, or have the car serviced. Be sure to keep the car filled with gas for any emergency.

In the Event of an Emergency

Imagine that someone in the group needs to call 911. Can all the group's members give clear directions to your friend's home, especially in an emergency? Is the house number visible from the street? Is the apartment building clearly marked? Are there landmarks or other descriptions that one can give to enable others to locate the address quickly and easily?

Captains should assign someone familiar with the area to take on the job of printing clear, concise directions to the person's house or apartment (include address, telephone number, and apartment number). This should be kept next to the phone along with the Share The Care Yellow Pages and numbers for police, fire, ambulance, and hospitals.

It would also be a good idea for the coordinator to send each member the same set of directions (especially if they are complicated or if some of the members are unfamiliar with the area) to keep with their copy of the Yellow Pages. It is very important that emergency information is at everyone's fingertips.

If there is an emergency, send someone outside the house or apartment building to direct EMS personnel to the right location.

When Everyone Is Using the Kitchen

The busiest room in Susan's apartment was the kitchen. So many of us would come over during the week to make or bring dinner for our buddy. This was all well and good, but we did have a few mishaps that you may want to avoid.

The Refrigerator

Susan's refrigerator was something to behold. It was filled with a United Nations of food types. Every imaginable country, nationality, and new age food trend could be found on its shelves: Myrna loved to bring spicy chicken with peanuts from the Chinese place on the corner. Barbara D. filled the fridge with tempting Italian treats from her mom's bakery. Joanne made pots of homemade chicken soup during the cold winter months. Cheryl brought tropical fruits and healthy greens and vegetables. Eileen B. delivered French cuisine from one of New York's best restaurants, and there was homemade pesto from Eileen M.

This was okay, but very often leftovers were stored away and forgotten only to be found at a later date when one of us cleaned out the refrigerator. Instead of being tasty lunches the next day, some dishes turned into moldy messes. You can avoid waste and confusion for all if the group follows some simple refrigerator tips:

- Label and date all food in the refrigerator or freezer (keep tape and a marker on top of the refrigerator to remind you).
- Don't bother saving small amounts of food that will never be eaten. Throw out the last tablespoon of mashed potatoes or pasta.
- Keep a running list of what needs to be replaced (attach to the front of the refrigerator or other specified place) for the group member assigned to do food shopping.
- If medications are stored in the refrigerator or freezer, put a note on the door so others are aware of it.

What under normal circumstances is just a messy kitchen can be a big problem to someone who is ill. It can also be a large annoyance to the caregivers when the person before them leaves a mess for them to clean up. If many of you are using your friend's kitchen, be extra considerate of your friend and your fellow group members.

- Put things back where they belong, even though it may take a while to get used to someone else's kitchen.
- Keep the kitchen clean by mopping up your spills right away.
- Don't leave dishes for the next person to wash.
- Fill the dishwasher and run it.
- Empty the dishwasher.
- Empty the garbage when you leave.

When Everyone Is Housekeeping

In a group caregiving situation, when many of you are visiting at different times, it will be helpful to your friend and the captains if you take care of small household jobs without being asked. When someone is ill, doing the smallest task is exhausting. Folding laundry, making the bed, watering the plants, and feeding the dog can be real chores. Be aware of what needs to be done and just do it, don't wait to be asked.

If there is some special larger job that needs attention, the captain should ask for a volunteer to do it. Orderly, clean, and cheery surroundings are important if you are recuperating at home.

I made kitchen curtains and covered Francine's chair seats . . . it made her so happy. (B.B.)

When Bob was in the hospital we gave his bedroom a fresh coat of paint, bought him a great blue bedspread (he loves blue), and hung some of his favorite prints that he never got around to framing. He was so pleased! I wish I had had a camera the day he arrived home! (C.L.)

How Things Work

This great idea for making household affairs run smoothly came from Dotty in California, who has had extensive experience working with groups:

Have someone write out instructions on the computer for each of the following areas that might be applicable. Put each page of instructions into a plastic sleeve and keep it on the appliance or in a binder marked "How Things Work" so people can refer to it as needed. The kitchen would probably be the best place for the binder.

- How the washer/dryer works
- Trash separation (paper, metal, glass etc); trash pick-up days
- Plumbing precautions
- Parking restrictions in the area
- Lawn-watering instructions
- Keys—location (good idea to label if there are several)
- Where to take the car for repairs
- How to defrost the fridge
- Location of toilet paper, paper towels, and other reserves
- Location of shovel, broom, mop/pail
- What and how much to feed the dog/cat/bird

When Everyone Is Shopping

One area where the group will need to coordinate its efforts will be keeping food and household supplies in stock. You don't want someone who is ill

Date: _____

SHOPPING LIST
(page 1)

Fill in size, brand, and amount needed next to each item.
This form can be filled in, saved, and edited online, then printed.

DAIRY		VEGETABLES	
Milk (whole, 1%, skim, lactose free, buttermilk, chocolate)		Potatoes (white, sweet)	
		Broccoli	
Cream		Peas	
Butter		Beans	
		Corn	
Margarine		Spinach	
Yogurt (low-fat, no-fat, flavors)		Tomatoes	
		Carrots	
Cheese		Celery	
Cottage cheese		Lettuce (type)	
		Onions (white, red)	
Eggs (egg substitute)		Cabbage (red, white)	
		Peppers	
BREAD - CEREAL - PASTA - RICE		Other:	
Bread (white, whole wheat, rye etc.)			
Breadsticks		**FRUITS**	
		Apples	
Crackers		Oranges	
Rice cakes		Grapefruit	
		Bananas	
Cold cereals		Grapes	
Hot cereals (instant/regular)		Cherries	
Pasta		Berries (strawberries/ blueberries/raspberries)	
		Peaches	
Rice (brown/white)		Plums	
		Nectarines	
POULTRY/MEATS - FISH		Melons	
Chicken		Lemons, limes	
Turkey		**FRUIT JUICE - FRESH - FROZEN - CANNED**	
Beef (cut)		Orange	
		Apple	
Pork		Grapefruit	
Veal		Cranberry	
		Other	
Fish			
Shellfish		**DRIED FRUIT - NUTS**	
		Fruits (raisins/prunes/apricots)	
Cold cuts		Nuts (salted/unsalted)	

SHOPPING LIST

Fill in size, brand and amount needed next to each item.

CANNED GOODS		PAPER GOODS	
Tomatoes		Toilet paper	
Tomato puree		Paper towels	
Tomato paste/sauce		Napkins	
Beans		Paper plates/cups	
Soups (low-salt, no-salt)		Other	
Tuna (packed in oil, water)		**HOUSEHOLD CLEANING SUPPLIES**	
Vegetables		Garbage bags	
Other		Trash bags	
COFFEE - TEA		Plastic storage/ freezer bags	
Coffee (regular, decaf)		Ammonia	
Instant coffee		Bleach	
Tea (regular, herbal, decaf)		Window cleaners	
Other		SOS/Brillo pads	
		Sponges/wipes	
CONDIMENTS		Hand soap	
Oil (olive, safflower)		Dishwashing liquid	
Vinegar		Dishwasher (powder, liquid, gel)	
Mustard		Woolite	
Ketchup		Detergent (powder, liquid)	
Mayonnaise		Fabric softener (liquid)	
Jams, jelly		Fabric softener (dryer sheets)	
Honey		Other	
Peanut butter (salt, no-salt)			
Pickles			
Olives			
Other			
SODA—WATER			
Bottled water			
Seltzer (plain or flavored)			
Cola (regular/diet /caffeine-free)			
Flavored sodas (regular/ caffeine-free)			
Iced tea			
Other			

DRUGSTORE ITEMS

ITEM	SIZE/BRAND/FLAVOR
Toothpaste	
Toothbrush	
Dental floss	
Mouthwash	
Deodorant (roll-on or spray)	
Sanitary napkins	
Tampons	
Shaving cream	
Razors	
Body lotion	
Face cream	
Makeup remover	
Contact lens supply (specific brand)	
Cleaner daily	
Cleaner weekly	
Saline solution	
Eyedrops	
Headache remedy	
Cold remedy	
Cotton balls	
Q-Tips	
Nail polish remover	
Shampoo	
Conditioner	
Hair spray	
Other items	

to run out of important items such as toilet paper, tissues, milk, bread, or juice.

To help your group get started we created a master shopping list and drugstore list. (They're reproduced here, or your group can create its own version.) One of the members can be assigned to ask the patient if he or she has any brand preferences and note them on the master list. This small consideration can mean a lot.

The master list can then be copied (make lots of them) and kept in a central place in the kitchen.

All this will be helpful to the person assigned to do the shopping for the week.

CHAPTER TWENTY

Getting Their Affairs in Order

In the event your friend is terminally ill and has no natural family or spouse (or is not on good terms with them), the job of helping get his or her affairs in order will fall to the caregivers. If you are the coordinator, the sooner this is handled the better. Does the group have all the information it needs should something happen to your friend? Do you know how to contact all out-of-town relatives and friends? Do you know where the safety deposit box key is kept? Do you know where the mortgage papers are located? Do you know the numbers of all the credit cards?

We have all heard stories of family and friends searching high and low for this information after someone has passed away and never locating it. You can avoid this situation by collecting the information now.

Collecting Vital Statistics and Locating Important Documents

Because your friend will need to trust the group and feel secure that any suggestions made by the caregivers are in his or her best interests, we recommend that two members who are very close to the patient handle this sensitive area, as well as the subjects of hospice care and final wishes, discussed later in this chapter.

We have tried to make collecting this much-needed information easier by including some charts (see pages 247 to 250). These charts not only serve as records but can assist in helping the group remember to cover as many points as possible. Feel free to add to these charts if need be, or devise your own.

The first thing to do is to make some specific, quiet time to sit with your friend, show him or her the charts, and start by asking for all the information requested on the list of Vital Statistics. Then move on to the Document Location Checklist. Last of all, do the List of Relatives/Friends. Keep the completed charts in a brightly colored folder marked "Vital Statistics and Document Location Checklist." Store the folder in a safe place (in the patient's home) where it can be referred to if needed.

Dealing with Legal Documents

As you are collecting information on the location of important documents you may discover that your friend does not have all of her or his affairs in order. This is the time to encourage your friend to put them in order as soon as possible.

- If there is no will, help your friend find an attorney and have one drawn up.
- If your friend cannot travel to the attorney's office, find a lawyer who will come to the house.
- At the same time, the patient can also appoint a power of attorney (if needed), deal with a Living Will and a Health Care Proxy, and determine an executor of the will.

The following is a brief description of some of the important documents your friend should have in order. An attorney can advise your friend in more detail.

Last Will and Testament

A will states the manner in which a person's estate (property: real estate, personal property, money, stocks, bonds, and other property rights) is disposed of upon the person's death. A will should also name an executor/executrix (the person responsible for administering the disposition of the estate) and a guardian, if minor children are involved.

There are many points and considerations (for example, real estate, debts, and bequests) that go into making these numerous and important decisions, and it is advisable that an attorney draw up a will for your friend. A handwritten will may be valid in only certain states and most probably will be subject to restrictions and circumstances. An attorney can advise the patient of the latest changes in the law and document the will to make sure all your friend's wishes will be carried out.

Regular Power of Attorney

This is a document that allows one person to appoint someone else (a relative, friend, or attorney) as a legal agent (called an "Attorney in Fact") to act on his or her behalf in situations concerning finances, property, or business. It can be drafted to expire when a specific business deal is completed or if the patient is declared incompetent, or it can be drafted so that it continues in full force and effect until specifically revoked.

Durable Power of Attorney

This is a legal document that authorizes one person to act on behalf of another in business and personal affairs even if the second person is declared legally incompetent.

THE MEDICAL DIRECTIVES

The following two documents (you need both to work together) can play a vital part in your friend's illness and treatment. A Living Will and Health Care Proxy are especially important if the patient does not want life prolonged by artificial means. As caregivers, it is important for you to know if your friend has already prepared these documents, known as medical directives. If he or she hasn't, encourage him or her to do so.

Your friend may need to carefully consider what he or she wants when filling out these documents. It may be helpful for your friend to discuss his or her thoughts with you if you are to be the health care agent (or proxy), and he or she may also need to discuss questions and desires with the physician, therapist, clergy, or attorney. Help to arrange these meetings for your friend as quickly as possible.

The Living Will

This is a written document that states an individual's wishes regarding life support and medical treatment in the event the person is not able at the end of life to make decisions or express wishes. This means one has the right to refuse (in advance) medical treatment and stipulate what care one does not want to receive. For example, people can choose whether they want cardiac resuscitation, mechanical respiration, tube feeding, antibiotics, and/or maximum pain relief if they have an incurable or irreversible mental or physical condition with no reasonable expectation of recovery.

The Health Care Proxy (or Durable Power of Attorney for Health Care)

This document allows a patient to appoint someone to make medical decisions for them if they are unable to do so, including decisions about life support. The Health Care Proxy is particularly useful because it appoints someone to speak for a person at any time that person is unable to make his or her own decisions, not only at the end of life.

Where Can You Get These Two Medical Directives?

Both can be purchased from most office supply stores. You can also visit http://www.partnershipforcaring.org or call 202-296-8071 for directives that comply with your state law. This organization also offers practical advice, legal information, and emotional support to help patients and families handle tough decisions about treatment at the end of life. Another source is Aging with Dignity at http://www.agingwithdignity.org or call 1-888-5-WISHES for their advance directives document, *Five Wishes.* The *Five Wishes* document is not valid in some states, so be sure to check the list on the Web site to see if your state recognizes it.

Where Should You Keep These Documents?

The signed original should be kept in the Vital Statistics and Document Location Folder in the patient's home. It is imperative that photocopies of the signed medical directives should go to

- All of the patient's doctors
- Real (biological) family members
- The attorney
- All those involved in the group, including free-floaters
- The Central Medical File
- The hospital file upon admission*

When someone is seriously ill, it is a relief to know these important matters have been handled. It is a great burden to have to deal with such issues at times of extreme stress. Sheila had some difficult moments because her mother had no Living Will and more than once when she was rushed to the hospital, Sheila had to sign a "do not resuscitate" order. Her mom was in her eighties and in critical condition. Without a doubt, she did not want to be put on any life-support systems should her heart or lungs give out (she had made her feelings known), yet it was painful to be confronted with the issue several times over.

Getting the Bills Paid

Has your friend considered what would happen should he or she become too ill to handle the tedious task of writing out the monthly bills (rent or mortgage, insurance, telephone, etc.)? One of you could suggest setting up an automatic bill payment service with the patient's bank.

First, make arrangements with all payors (Social Security, Disability, etc.) to have incoming checks to the patient deposited directly into your friend's bank account. Contact the bank for details on its particular

---

* See chapter 14, "Ten Steps to Making a Hospital Stay as Painless as Possible," for a discussion of what to take to the hospital.

monthly bill-payment service. You can usually establish this service by phone or by filling out an application at the bank.

Some of the information you will need to set this service up will include: name, account number, a list of all signers on the account, and a list of individuals or companies to be paid, including address and account number for each. Additions and deletions can be made to this list at any time.

Health Insurance Forms and Procedures

Handling health insurance forms and procedures is a time-consuming job that requires persistence, patience, and good record keeping. If there is another member employed by the same company where the patient worked, the coordinator could ask that member to assist on a permanent basis in this area. Susan was fortunate in that she had two such women at her office, Joanne and Myrna, who were able to plead her cause and enlist her company's support in getting Susan the most from her health-care benefits.

We found that it is extremely important for the person with this job to have the insurance booklet explaining the coverage provided. Even with this booklet it is often confusing or difficult to figure out what is and is not covered, especially when dealing with a major illness. Insurance companies do have 800 numbers to call for help. Use them as often as you need to.

Some advice we can offer to the person taking on the job:

- Never allow health insurance to expire. Make sure your friend's bills are paid on time and in full. If insurance is lost it might be extremely difficult to reinstate or replace.
- Keep good records of everything; make copies of documentation of all claims, bills, receipts, and correspondence.
- Keep a record of claims—pending, paid, and submitted.
- When calling the insurance company, be clear and prepared with all vital information. If you have a problem you can get a lot further if you remain calm and try to work out a solution. We have found from personal experience that getting hysterical over insurance company red tape really gets you nowhere.
- Be sure to get the name and title of the person you speak to at the insurance

company. Write these things down, along with the day you called. This way you can avoid needless repetition every time you call.

- Fill in needed information on the claim forms *ahead of time* (name, address, date of birth, sex, medical insurance group numbers, etc.) and have the patient sign them. This way you can submit bills immediately.

Life Insurance and Disability Insurance

When someone is seriously or suddenly ill, the first thing that comes to mind is health insurance. However, other kinds of insurance may be equally important. In most life insurance policies, there is a new benefit called "living benefit." This benefit provides that if the illness is terminal, the person who is ill can pull all life insurance benefits forward, so that instead of leaving the money to someone else, he or she can draw on it to help pay for medical costs or other necessary expenses.

For young or middle-aged people, disability insurance can make a huge difference. Remember, health insurance pays only the doctors and health institutions that provide care, but disability insurance provides that while people are ill or recovering from an accident or illness, especially a long-term one, they will still have their homes, some recreation, and the lifestyle they were used to before they became ill. Most companies do provide employees with some form of disability insurance. Be sure to find out if your friend has it, and keep up with the claims. It can be the difference between hope and despair.

Acquire a list of all the pertinent insurance policies and follow the coverage guidelines for them as well.

Hospice Care

At the same time you are assisting your sick friend in dealing with legal issues and specific advance medical directives, you might bring up the subject of hospice care* and final wishes, especially if your friend is suffering

---

* See "Helpful Associations" (List of Resources) in the back of the book for contact information for several hospice organizations.

with a terminal illness. Though it is a difficult conversation to initiate, it is realistically an important one to have.

Does your friend understand what hospice care means and has he or she talked about it with the doctor? The general guideline for admittance into a hospice program is written certification by a doctor (the patient's own physician or a hospice doctor) that a patient is believed to have a life expectancy of six months or less. Importantly, the patient has the right to accept or deny this kind of care.

Tell your friend that the ideas behind hospice care are the acceptance of dying as part of life and the exclusion of all treatments, machines, and medications meant to prolong life. A hospice program provides care that is comfort oriented (pain management and practical nursing support and emotional support) for the patient *in the home*. And it provides very important emotional support for family and friends as well.

If, for some reason, your friend is unable to discuss hospice care with a doctor, as the caregivers you may need to do so. (We also found it a good idea for the group to communicate with the doctor when there is a change in the patient's condition that may signal a turning point. In Susan's case it was when she no longer was able to stand and took to her bed permanently.)

Several of you can visit the hospice the doctor refers you to or visit others in your area and talk to the staff and find out about their programs and services. Do you find them compassionate and willing to help? We strongly recommend doing this research before it is actually needed and you are emotionally stretched to your limits as caregivers.

Final Wishes

When someone is very ill, discussing final wishes is a calm recognition of the inevitable. Many people have no idea what they would answer to the questions listed below. But when they start thinking and talking about them with people who love them, they begin to feel better and somehow relieved.

You may even discover that you and your friend are brought closer together by having touched on many of these areas that are filled with emotion.

When these details are decided upon, your friend will be able to have his or her final wishes carried out and there will be less confusion, expense, doubts, and distress for those left behind.

- Who should be contacted (out-of-town friends, relatives, business associates, insurance companies, associations, etc.)? *
- What kind of funeral (memorial) service does your friend want?
- Does he or she want cremation? Burial?
- Does he or she have a cemetery plot? Where is the deed (you will need it)? †
- Does your friend want to be buried in a special dress or suit? Put these clothes and all accessories and religious articles in a designated place.
- Does your friend have a written list of the possessions he or she wants to give to specific friends or relatives?
- Do you know biographical information (that could be included in an obituary)?
- Does your friend have any other special requests (readings, songs, poems, etc.)?

Two caregivers recall some specific final requests:

Years ago I remember a very special woman (a business associate) who was suffering from cancer. When she died a wonderful champagne party for all her friends and business associates was held at her request. It was a most amazing party . . . everyone had a great time laughing and telling stories of times they had shared with their friend. It was a joyous occasion and a reflection of who she was in life. (R.F.)

Recently an old friend whom I hadn't seen in ages told me he was HIV positive and had been doing a lot of thinking about his final wishes. He decided that he wanted cremation and his ashes divided up into seven packages and sent to seven friends living in various wonderful, magical places all over the globe. He wanted his friends to scatter his ashes in the places he had visited, had happy times, and loved for different reasons. I was very moved and thought this is a very amazing way to celebrate his life in his death. (L.T.)

* See Vital Statistics (List of Relatives/Friends, page 250).
† See the Document Location Checklist (page 248).

This form can be filled in, saved, and edited online, then printed.	Date: _____

SHARE THE CARE

VITAL STATISTICS

Name:	
Address:	
E-mail address:	
Telephone:	
Business address:	
Business telephone:	
Occupation/title:	
Date of birth:	
Place of birth:	
Citizenship papers:	
Passport number:	
Social Security Number:	
War Veteran Serial Number:	
Father's name:	
Father's place of birth:	
Mother's maiden name:	
Mother's place of birth:	
Religion:	

| This form can be filled in, saved, and edited online, then printed. | Date: _____ |

S H A R E   T H E   C A R E

DOCUMENT LOCATION CHECKLIST

(page 1)

DOCUMENT	LOCATION
Birth certificate (or other proof of age)	
Will	
Power of Attorney	
Living Will	
Health Care Proxy	
Organ donation card	
Social Security card	
Marriage license	
Prenuptial agreements	
Divorce papers	
Trust agreements	
Citizenship papers	
Passport	
Veteran's discharge papers	
Safety deposit box (bank)	
Safety deposit key	
Mortgage papers/deeds	
Car papers/insurance	
Bank accounts	
checking	
savings	
CDs	
Stock/bonds	
IRAs	
Keoghs	

This form can be filled in, saved and edited online, then printed.	Date: _____

SHARE THE CARE

DOCUMENT LOCATION CHECKLIST (page 2)

DOCUMENT	LOCATION
Credit cards and #'s	
Income tax receipts	
Income tax returns	
Pension	
Life insurance	
Health insurance	
Supplementary health insurance	
Disability insurance	
Medicare	
Medicaid	
Cemetery (include address)	
Burial plot (lot and grave number)	
Vault	
Final wishes	

Date: _____

SHARE THE CARE

LIST OF RELATIVES/FRIENDS

NAME	RELATIONSHIP	ADDRESS/PHONE/E-MAIL

PART 4

Keeping the Group (and Yourself) Going

CHAPTER TWENTY-ONE

Being with Someone Who Is Seriously Ill

We've talked about all things you can *do* to help. But sometimes the thing people need from you the most is the hardest thing of all . . . to just *be* with them. It's easier to run around doing things, keeping busy and solving specific problems, than it is to just be there with their pain, their fear, their anger, their guilt.

Listening

Listening, without interruption, can be difficult for those of us who are "talkers." But listening has its rewards. You may truly learn what it is like to be in someone else's place. You may gain remarkable insights from people facing their mortality. Only one thing is certain. If you allow your friend time to fully express himself, it will bring you closer. There are many things you will never have to do in a caregiver group, but listening is not one of them.

Learn to listen. Try to be patient when people tell you the same thing over and over. Remember, the information they're dealing with is so shocking that it may require a lot of processing for it to sink in. No matter how understanding their doctors are, no one in the medical establishment can give them what you can . . . time. Listening can be a form of healing because it lets them come to terms with what is happening and it lets them know someone cares.

Their reality is shifting rapidly. Sometimes they go through psychological changes in a matter of months that would normally take years. If you don't listen, you won't know what's appropriate at any given moment.

Pay attention to what they say. If they say they can't breathe, listen. If they say they don't want to go to the hospital, listen. If they say they're claustrophobic and can't go in an MRI machine, take them seriously. Also listen to their little requests. If they want a certain new music selection to make them feel better, listen. They're already feeling like they're losing control. If you don't listen, they will feel this even more.

Listening to someone who is very ill or dying may lead you into some serious re-examination of your own priorities in life. It can make you come to appreciate what you have or what you are doing.

Because I had had cancer ten years ago (Hodgkin's disease), my question to myself was, Can I handle this? How far have I come in my own emotional healing? I had helped a number of people in the past, but not a truly dear friend who was my age. But because of the group, I was able to have a conversation with my friend about the possibility that she might die from her lymphoma. I was touched that she confided in me and we had an opportunity to discuss our fears, hopes, and desire for ultimate peace. (G.A.)

Talking

You'd be surprised how far a gentle word can go with people who are suffering. When they accomplish something, however small, acknowledge them. When they're wheeled off to surgery, tell them you'll be there when they get back. Tell them how well they're doing with their diet, their physical therapy, their giving up smoking, and so forth. If they are losing some of their physical abilities, conversation may be the thing that gets them through their days. If they feel they are losing control of their lives, they want to be kept informed. Don't leave them out of the decisions they can help make. They are probably very worried about how you are doing. Talk to them about how you're feeling.

However, there are some things you should never say to a person who is very ill. When they ask how you are, *don't say,* "Oh, I'm fine. I mean, compared to what you're going through, I have no problems." This makes them feel that they must be in really bad shape. Be honest with them about your life. They want to hear your problems, if only to forget about their own for a while.

When they just found out about their fourth surgery, *don't say,* "It's going to be okay. Don't worry. This time, I know it's going to be okay." If they've been getting progressively sicker, they're afraid to think they're going to be okay because if it doesn't turn out that way they're setting themselves up for a terrible disappointment. It's better to say "I'm here. I'll be with you, whatever happens."

When they've accepted the fact that they're not going to get better, *don't say,* "What do those doctors know? You'll be on your feet in no time." The human spirit has an amazing capacity to deal with what is and try to come to terms with it. If they have come to terms with their illness and possibly imminent death, you can't expect them to put up with your fears and indulge you in your own denial. If you can't face the facts with them, let someone else in the group do it.

Being Sensitive

When it's your time to be with the person who is ill, stop and think about how he or she might be feeling. If your friend is on a macrobiotic diet and you're craving a burger and fries, leave time to eat before you go to visit. If your friend just got bad news about another surgery, don't talk about your dance class. If he or she has just had a fight with a son or daughter about their grades, don't bring up the fact that your son or daughter just won a scholarship to Harvard.

If your friend has a doctor's appointment in the morning and is feeling apprehensive, don't babble on about the thunderstorm that is due to hit in the morning. Remember, you have a whole support group you can call on if you aren't able to deal with your friend's concerns.

Be sensitive if your friend has lost or is in the process of losing some of his or her physical abilities. Don't stare at a neck brace or a sling. Don't overstay your welcome if your friend looks tired.

It was a very hard thing to watch Susan go from clicking across the pavement in her high-heeled shoes to walking painfully with a cane to using a walker to her first reluctant ride in a wheelchair to the day when she realized she would never leave her bed. But it was inspiring to know that all through that long and difficult journey there was always someone there, encouraging her, acknowledging her bravery and her triumphs, holding her hand, telling her she wasn't alone.

The Power of Touch

When people are seriously ill, one of the things that often happens is that people stop touching them, just when they need a hug, a kiss, a hand, or a pat on the shoulder the most. People in hospitals are rarely touched, though research has shown that touch can enhance the healing process. Older people who are never touched seem to wither up and die, while those who have lots of physical contact from family and friends seem stronger and more vibrant. So even if you're frightened of how weak or fragile a person may seem, go ahead and put your arms around them. Wash her hair or give him a shave. Offer a manicure or a massage. And don't underestimate the healing power of touch.

Sheila recalls:

> On my visits to see my mom in the nursing home, one of the things I was able to do for her when she was totally immobile and bedridden was to bring her "Sheila's Beauty Shop." I would start by giving her lots of hugs and kisses. Then I would wash her face, brush her hair, and spray her with some fresh-smelling cologne. Sometimes I would set her hair with soft rollers. Then I got out her body lotion and massaged her back, arms, hands, legs, and ended with a foot massage. I did my best to freshen her senses and without fail she was always more relaxed and peaceful when I left. I felt really good about doing this for her as it was all I *could* do.

Don't Treat Your Friend Like an Alien

When two or more of you are with the person who is ill, be careful not to talk only to each other and leave the patient out. He or she might have cancer, ALS, or AIDS or be in a wheelchair, but that doesn't mean he or she can't think or talk.

Often visitors talk about a sick friend in the third person while that individual is there in the room. They say things like "Well, Susan's going to rest soon. She's awfully tired today" or "Barbara's going into the hospital tomorrow, so we better pack her bag." People do this because they think it's sparing the patient, but it usually has the opposite effect. The sick person already feels isolated from the rest of the world. Maybe he's had to leave a job. Some of her friends might have deserted her. Talking *about* them instead of *with* them makes them feel even more isolated. It's better to include them in the conversation and talk directly to them when they are there, even if it's a difficult subject.

Build Your Time with Them into Your Schedule

Don't think you can squeeze being part of a caregiver group into your life without some planning. This is a real commitment and has to be given its own place. Handle whatever else is going on in your life so that when you are with your friend you're really *with* him or her. If an emergency arises in your own family and you're feeling overwhelmed, get somebody else to cover for you. If you have a deadline at the office or a project and you're preoccupied, don't try to help your friend figure out an insurance claim. If you've never known the meaning of "quality time," this is a good time to find out.

Know When to Not Be There

Just as important as being with your friend is knowing when to *not* be with your friend. He might need to be alone. She might be tired from too many group members running in and out. Most important, he or she might need something from someone else in the group or from a real family member and it may be something you can't give. Don't deprive your friend of what that person has to give by rushing in and filling all the spaces. Leave room for the other people your friend needs.

Find a Way to Be with Them That Works for You

When someone has a very serious illness or one that goes on for a long time, it's easy for the illness to become an obsession and to take up all the space in a person's life. Just as you must know when to listen, you should try to learn when you should pull your friend out of obsessing about operations, drugs, and doctors.

One way is to find something you can do together. It will help your friend to feel that life still has meaning, and it will help you when being with your friend is just too painful. This was an issue that came up for Cappy:

I was one of the people who had a very hard time just "being with" Susan. Hanging out, sitting still, and allowing unstructured time weren't the things I did well in the first place, but hanging out with someone who was dying was impossible. I was terrified.

So I would *do* everything imaginable: bring her books on healing, suggest ways for her to stop smoking, do vegetarian cooking together, anything but just *be*.

At first Susan appreciated my madcap energy. She said I made her forget her illness for a while. But as her battle with cancer became tougher and tougher, my high energy, optimism, and enduring faith that she would win out over death began to wear thin. But it was then that Susan and I discovered a way to be together that would change both our lives. We began to write a screenplay called *Susan's Funny Family.*

We worked on it for two years, up until her death, spending countless hours talking about the amazing family of friends and eventually about the mystery of death, the miracle of life. It became our special journey, a journey that would take everything I had to give, wound me deeply, and ultimately heal both of us in ways I could never have imagined. It became her reason for living and my way to come to grips with sickness, death, and human limitations.

Find a Healing Way to Be Together as a Group

More than likely there will be a time when you all will have an opportunity to come together to take part in some healing or spiritual practice. This will bond you even tighter and allow you to understand what you are doing on a profound new level. Your loved one may request the group do something for him or her. Or someone in the group may offer to teach or lead everyone in a practice that would be beneficial to you all. Take advantage of these gifts as they come your way. Many, many groups have shared how they have healed with each other whether in their meetings, during an important milestone, or in their day-to-day work. We encourage your group to cultivate its spiritual side in whatever way feels appropriate. Be open and trusting that you will find what is right for your group.

Hands-On Healing

Norma, who lived in California, suffered from liver and gallbladder cancer. Her group of twenty-two consisted mainly of family, friends, and fellow teachers. Maureen, one of her group members, shared the Hands-on Healing experience some of them incorporated after the end of the first meeting:

> The night we held the meeting Norma was able to participate in the first part and retired to the bedroom while the second part took place. Once the meeting was officially over, one of the teachers discreetly asked if there were others who would like to join her to lay hands on Norma in the other room. There were five or six of us and as Norma lay on the bed, one person held her hand, another stroked her forehead, someone touched her leg, another her foot, as we prayed that she be healed and said the Our Father in soft wisps of voices around her. I have done this before, but this time I was praying that this would be the one time that we could really be the conduits for total physical healing. Just as we ended our prayer, Norma's sister-in-law walked in and said she had come with the intent of

calming her since she thought she'd be upset because her boyfriend was late in coming to pick her up. Norma said that she felt she had just been calmed and felt truly relaxed.

A Healing Circle

This information came from Marion, a friend of Lisa, who had a diagnosis of multiple myeloma.

The idea for a healing circle originated with me and another friend as we both lived in different parts of the country and groped for a way to be of help to Lisa, who was on the West Coast. We now have some happy news to report: over the last two years Lisa has undergone a stem cell transplant and joyfully it was a success and she is now in remission.

The healing circle was simply done by setting a time (10–10:30 p.m. EST—and however that translated all over the world) each night for everyone to pray/meditate at the exact same moments together. It was up to each person to decide for how much of the half hour to participate. We continued nightly, usually for one to two weeks, depending on where Lisa was in her treatment/recovery. We tried to overlap with all the days of her chemo, for example. Then as the treatment wound down, I would remind people we were going to close that round (I didn't want people to begin to forget or get tired of participating). We ran the circle via e-mail reminders at least five times on and off over six months.

Lisa was quite aware of this effort. And she expressed a lot of gratitude and had some tears over it. She did express feeling its power in some indescribable way. Perhaps just knowing how much we were all there for her and wanting her to get well and live again and be able to be all the things she is to us all—maybe that was what she "got" from it. Of course, as things got better and better in terms of her good response to treatment, she became convinced that the healing circle was an important part of her recovery.

People were free to say whatever prayer they wanted. Most evenings I simply prayed at my puja (a Sanskrit word for "altar"), as I follow an Indian-based spiritual path. Other days I said a very special fairly long prayer in Sanskrit that is said every day in certain Indian ashrams. I have found this prayer to be very powerful in general in my life in terms of giving me guidance. For others not accustomed to praying, I suggested that they simply "send positive thoughts" of love and wellness to Lisa by thinking about her. Several Jewish friends recited a special blessing for healing (Mi Sheh Berach or Refuah Shlomah). Some asked me for guidance about what to do and many seemed to figure out the "right thing" on their own.

Healing at Home

When illness struck, Cappy called on all the therapists and healers in her life to play a role. One of those healers was a man named Richard whom Cappy had met just months before she became ill. When Cappy finally returned to New York permanently, Richard started coming to the city to see her every week. It was a long trip in for him, nearly three hours each way. Using a combination of touch, crystal, aromatherapy, color healing, meridian, and chakra work his visits left her feeling incredibly happy and peaceful. Then, at Cappy's urging many in the Brain Trust started booking sessions with Richard as well. One day a week, Cappy's apartment became a "healing center" for everyone. We booked appointments through a "healer captain." One after the other we'd show up to visit with her before or after our session, depending on how tired she was.

Cappy truly loved having initiated these healing sessions. She always had a great concern for her friends and it was her way of getting us to bond with each other. We found these times a way to become involved in Cappy's healing and reinforce our connection to each other as a group. Richard's powerful work helped us to focus our awareness on living in the "now" moment. This left us more relaxed and centered so we could continue to juggle our lives and group commitments.

Building a Labyrinth

The group known as The Swimmers (after the name of a folk song that has to do with transitions: "swimming to the other side") consisted of fifty men and women, including two teens. One of their most amazing accomplishments was to lay the brickwork to create a labyrinth so their dear friend Sharon, who suffered from breast cancer, could walk it twice daily and later be wheeled through it. Her husband, Brian, explains.

> I e-mailed a couple people in the group about creating a labyrinth and almost instantaneously a group of volunteers appeared. So when we started it in the fall of 2002 all of the group members worked on it. Sharon even helped carry many of the paving bricks. We hired some high school students for a day as well. I did most of the actual laying of the bricks and it was finished in June when my father was visiting. He was able to help run the masonry saw and this was a good grandfather, father, son experience. The labyrinth was based on the famous Chartres Cathedral labyrinth in France. My son Marcus and I spent time with graphics programs and spreadsheets to design and plan it.
>
> When it was finished Sharon shared it with many people. She was a member of a Spirituality Group, a group of women who had met for many years to share their joys and concerns and to walk with each other on their spiritual paths. Once Sharon was in a wheelchair, "Swimmers" would drop in at appointed times during the day, and at least once a day the walk with the wheelchair was a journey along the labyrinth path.
>
> If others wanted to create something like this, they should know it was a rather large undertaking and cost four thousand dollars. So I am not sure how accessible what we did is to others. We also had the space and the tractor that made it possible. There are examples of people mowing the path into their lawns, so there are less intensive alternatives.

Phowa Guided Meditation

Susan, a member of The Swimmers (and a neurologist and certified meditation instructor) introduced Phowa to everyone and led weekly guided imagery and meditation sessions for Sharon and those in the group who chose to attend. Upon her passing, twenty-five people came to sit with Sharon. It was a very powerful experience. Susan explains how it works.

Phowa, you might say, is a Tibetan Buddhist meditation practice that requires no specific beliefs of the participant. This makes it ideal for practice with a group of mixed religious faiths, and it works also with people who have no designated faith. The practice has components of visualization of an embodiment of truth, wisdom, and compassion; meditation on aspects that need purification or forgiveness; visualization of the purification and forgiveness; visualization of merging with the energy of the embodiment of wisdom and compassion, with the awareness that this is our true nature. Another thing that makes it especially powerful is that it is taught as a practice for life; one that if we master during life makes our dying peaceful, so people are practicing for themselves too. For more specific information, see *Facing Death and Finding Hope: A Guide to the Emotional and Spiritual Care of the Dying.**

Creating a Healing Altar

Some of us in Cappy's group got great support out of creating and maintaining a Healing Altar.† It can be a transformational experience for all involved. A home altar is like having your own little temple or place for reflection right in your own room. You can to build one easily using religious books, objects, or statues. Or you can use things that come entirely from nature: seashells, rocks, starfish, driftwood, bird nests, feathers, sage, and flowers. It can be a mixture of things from different cultures and times. What is most important in creating a Healing Altar is the *intention* behind it.

To start, have your loved one select what objects they would like to have included. Perhaps photos of when they were in good health, photos of loved ones, a votive candle, roses in a variety of colors, leaves, beautiful stones, a seahorse, rose quartz crystals, bells, or pieces of beach glass. It could also include tiny animals, stars, a fountain, or postcards. If it is for a child, they may want special dolls or stuffed animals. Add a child's artwork, jewelry, or a personal treasure like an old harmonica. Perhaps it might contain a written message, poetry, a letter, or an inspiring saying. Or a rock

* See Helpful Books, page 322.
† See Special Interest Books, page 324.

with the word *love* carved into it. Maybe it is a little gondola from that magical trip to Venice or a bowl of fresh oranges. The inspiration is up to the individual. Situate the altar on a table, shelf, or windowsill where the patient can see it from bed or a wheelchair, and arrange all the objects on a pretty scarf, tablecloth, or scrap of material.

Once the altar has been arranged you need to bless it with good intentions. This would be a nice thing to do with a small group. Start by lighting a candle and some incense if you like. Ring a bell and ask everyone to join hands in a circle or fold them in prayer position or hold them over their hearts (whatever feels right). Then, going in a clockwise direction have everyone say some words, prayers, or sing to the healing of the patient while the others visualize them smiling, happy, and in good health. That's it.

Every day, the altar will remind the patient of the beautiful thoughts and intentions behind it and she or he will be able to take pleasure in the objects on it and their specific meanings. The candle can be lit every day and a prayer (or other words) repeated to reinforce the intention.

A Comforting Creation

Maureen from Norma's Share The Care group described a special Memory Book one member put together.

> Someone among us who was very creative made a scrapbook/photo album to treasure. It contains photographs from the first meeting; feelings written down by everyone at the beginning and toward the end of the meeting; everyone's reasons for wanting to be a member of the group; plus an abundance of cards and notes Norma received throughout her illness. It was a work of art that Norma could look through, over and over again to remind herself of all the love with which she was surrounded. Priceless.

CHAPTER TWENTY-TWO

What-Ifs, Do's, and Don'ts

This section contains short takes on a number of issues that may come up during the life of your caregiver family. Some contain practical advice based on lessons we learned the hard way (for example, "Do Break the Problem Up into Little Pieces," "What If There's a Big Crisis?" and "Don't Be Late").

Some contain psychological advice we learned through trial and error, intuition, and advice from experts (for example, "Do Learn How to Say No as Well as Yes," "What If Your Friend Wants to Talk About Dying?" and "Don't Let Them Project Their Fears onto You").

Obviously, not every issue will apply to your group, but we hope that many of them will be helpful.

What If . . .

There's a Big Crisis?

Don't try to handle it alone. Divide the tasks up into categories.

PERSON #1

Have one person there just to be with, talk to, and comfort the patient. In a big crisis, small things like having someone to calmly explain what's going on, hold a hand, carry a wallet or purse, or keep track of personal belongings can make a huge difference.

PERSON #2

Have one person to deal with the immediate logistics—calling the doctor, arranging for transportation to the hospital, locking up the house or apartment of the person going to the hospital.

PERSON #3

Have one person to deal with miscellaneous backup—going to the drugstore, picking up or delivering X-rays or test results, getting the phone chain going so other group members know what's going on, and most important, taking care of the other two caregivers (getting lunch, making a phone call to a husband or wife or daughter, arranging for relief people to take over from persons 1 and 2).

What If...

There's a Small Crisis but It's Big to the Person Who Is Ill?

People who are seriously ill are often ultrasensitive and tend to see every problem, no matter how big or how small, as another crisis. There's a delicate balance between knowing when to be very gentle and totally understanding and when to make light of something.

When Susan's shower went from cold to scalding hot without warning (at a time when she was recovering from hip surgery), there was a great danger she could move suddenly and fall. She was very upset (understandably), and we reacted immediately to get it fixed. But when her air conditioner broke in the middle of the summer, she was just as hysterical, even though this was obviously not a life-threatening situation.

Often, people who are seriously ill have had so many crises that they tend to lump together everything from the mild to the serious to the catastrophic. It's up to you to distinguish among them. Mild crises require understanding and attention but can be dealt with without turning yourself inside out. A little humor could even help. Serious crises that are not immediately threatening (like the shower) still require fast attention. Big crises require immediate attention and probably more than one group member.

What If . . .

Your Friend Wants to Try an Alternative, Unproven, or Exotic Cure?

What if your friend wants to try apricot pits or black paste? Or wants to meditate at three A.M., see an Indian guru, eat only brown rice, or move to the Caribbean?

One of the biggest lessons we learned in taking care of Susan was that cancer, like life, is mercurial, mysterious, and complex; that there are no simple answers, and that no one knows why some people get it and die, while others get it, go into remission, and live out their lives.

We learned that no one system or idea works for everyone, that doctors are not gods, and that the will to live does seem to play a part in people's getting well. We read about and met people who convinced us that they had cured themselves of the disease. We also met people desperately running from one guru to another trying to find an answer when modern medicine failed them.

Many of the diseases we are facing today have stumped the scientists, the doctors, and the medical establishment. To some degree, people who have been afflicted have to figure out a lot on their own. So, if meditation helps them get through a radiation treatment or surgery, it should be encouraged. If visualization can ease their pain, by all means be supportive. People who are facing serious illness and know they are probably going to die journey to a place that most of us cannot enter yet. All we can do is try not to judge.

What If . . .

You're Feeling Strangely Detached?

Sometimes, during the course of someone's illness, you may have strong feelings of detachment, as if you were not a part of the scene around you. It's not unusual to feel this way, particularly when a crisis hits and your caregiving duties intensify. You feel like "I'm in a movie and all this just isn't happening," but unfortunately it is.

We experienced such a "lost day." While talking to her doctor one morning on Fire Island, Susan discovered that she was to have another surgery and she had to leave the island on the next boat. We called one of the group members in the city and made arrangements for that person to meet her when she got home.

After we put Susan on the ferry to the mainland that morning, the rest of the day held a total sense of unreality. We have no idea what we said, did, or thought. We wandered along the beach, and at about four in the afternoon found ourselves in the next community eating frozen yogurt and feeling as if we had been frozen in time. We didn't even remember walking there.

If you experience such detachment or depression, we urge you to be gentle and understanding with yourself. These are real feelings. If at all possible, don't do anything that requires alertness or precision. Let someone else do the driving. Let it pass.

What If . . .

You Show Up and Your Friend Wants to Be Alone?

It may be hard to conceive that someone who is going through a devastating illness can turn away the comfort of your company, but it will happen. Sometimes such people can talk only to other people who have their disease. Sometimes the "healthy" world seems very foreign to them. Sometimes they are just plain exhausted.

But the hardest thing for those who are caregivers may be the realization that the patient is feeling strong and is coping with the disease; they don't want you there because you are not as strong as they are, because you have more fear than they do, because they know you can't or won't talk about death with them, or because they know you will get too emotional and they don't want to be emotional that evening.

If it happens, just accept it. Take the time that has been freed up and do something for yourself or for someone else in the group. Don't put yourself down; don't force your kindness on your friend. At some other time your friend will probably tell you what he or she was feeling and why he or she did not want to be with you.

What If...

Money Becomes an Issue?

At some point during the time your Share The Care group is in operation, money may become an issue.

Even if the person who is ill is fortunate enough to be well provided for, there are certain out-of-pocket expenses that are hard for caregivers to avoid—carfare, lunch, groceries, trips to the cleaners or the drugstore, gasoline, and many others. When a person is in pain or frightened or panicked, it may seem petty to consider the cost of a cab ride.

If money is not a problem for you, you may feel fine about paying for these things. But if it becomes a problem, you must speak up. People who are seriously ill are often overly fearful that the money will run out (even if they have enough) and they may unwittingly take advantage.

At Susan's, we had a bowl with Susan's money in it for things like groceries and laundry, and whoever was visiting just took what they needed from the bowl. If the money situations of the people in your group are greatly varied, you might put a sign on the bowl saying people can contribute to the slush fund if they'd like.

However you do it, make sure it gets handled. Don't let it get in the way of caring for someone you love.

What If...

Your Friend Wants to Talk About Dying?

When people who are sick want to talk about death and dying, it isn't always out of fear and it isn't because they are morbid and depressed. It is often because that is the subject they are interested in. That is what is happening to them. There comes a time when they are no longer really involved in the world of the living. They seem to drift off and you may feel you are fighting an invisible force to keep them here.

If it's too painful for you to discuss death, find someone in the group who is comfortable with such a conversation, or find a therapist, hospice worker, or support group for your friend. At the back of this book, there is a reading list with books that can help.

Don't . . .

Say That Everything's Going to Be Okay If It Isn't

There may come a time when people have accepted how sick they are and you haven't. At this time, if you say "It's going to be okay," they may explode at you. They need you to be real with them, perhaps even to face death with them or tell them it's okay for them to leave. You may come right up against your own fear of death, and you may need some counseling yourself. Get it, or you will be no good to your friend or to yourself.

Do . . .

Keep Your Sense of Humor

Even in dire circumstances there is always something worth smiling about, and laughter is one of the most healing responses we have. Even the medical community acknowledges that there may be real physical benefits in laughter.

One way to keep a sense of humor is to stay in the present moment. If the person you are caring for has to have a scary test or treatment, try not to live it or let him or her live it six times before it actually happens.

Also, try to keep a broader perspective. No one knows what will happen to any one of us the next day or hour or minute, so the more we can all enjoy the present the better off we'll be. If you can't cheer the patient up, bring in a group member who has the gift of humor, and be around people who make you laugh. Watch a funny TV program or movie or read something you find amusing. You'll see. A sense of humor makes even more sense when things are tough.

Don't...

Wear Out Your Friend Because She's Always Available

When people who were very active are forced to stay home because of illness, often what happens is that others around them discover how nice it is to have quality time with the people they love. And, because people who are ill are always available, it may be tempting for group members to drop by more often than they are scheduled to.

If your group has ten or more people in it, it's easy to see that the person who is ill could have too much excitement, too much energy, too many people around. Susan was a good listener, and when she first quit her job to stay home, she always had people dropping in, telling her their stories and their troubles. At other times, three or four of us would show up at once and decide to all have dinner together. It was tempting to turn these visits into a party. At one point, Susan had to tell us that in spite of how much she enjoyed our visits, we had become too much for her.

Do...

Keep Your Friend Involved in Life

It's very easy when you're caring for someone who is seriously ill over a long period of time to think of that person as identified with an illness. It's almost as if such people *are* their disease. Yet often people at the end of their physical lives have a great deal to give, mentally and spiritually. So don't stop sharing your dreams, your hopes, your own problems. Don't stop asking for their advice. They need to be allowed to do what they can, and their wisdom may amaze you.

Don't...

Let Your Friend Treat You Badly and Get Away with It

It's hard to get angry at someone who's dying or someone who's in constant pain. But if you don't express your feelings, even your anger, you are denying your friend a real relationship, separating her or him from real life, and doing great damage to yourself. You may need to say, "Stop screaming at me! I did not give you this cancer. It is not my fault you are sick. I love you and I am doing the best I can, but I can't be here for you if you treat me badly."

Do . . .

Own Your Love

Your friend needs to hear you say "I love you," but it's just as important to you to acknowledge how much you love your friend. When the patient, or someone in the group, tells you you did great, let the compliment in. We're all so quick to acknowledge how imperfect we are, how we could have done more or better. What you're doing is very special, very important, very difficult. Own your goodness.

Don't . . .

Let Them Project Their Fears onto You

It was seven A.M. Cappy had spent the night at Susan's and was in the kitchen, making coffee. Susan walked in with her walker and totally out of the blue began to lecture Cappy about how much money Cappy spent. She was certain Cappy would end up in the street with no money and no one to take care of her in old age.

Cappy didn't know it at the time, but Susan was projecting . . . that is, she was taking a fear of hers and trying to place it on someone else. People who are very ill are often afraid that the money will run out and no one will take care of them. With the size of doctor and hospital bills today, this is understandable. But this can happen even if they have all the money they need. Susan had a large disability plan and really didn't have to worry about money. Irrational fears often surface when people confront illness and dying. So instead of telling you how frightened *they* are, they say they are frightened for *you*.

If a person who is ill begins to lecture you, especially if what she is saying makes no sense, realize she may be talking about herself.

Do . . .

Let Them Do What They Still Can

When someone has been struggling with disabilities, pain, and physical impairment, little accomplishments can be triumphs. Let your friend have the dignity of doing what he or she can. When Susan was in an alternative care clinic in the Bahamas, she could hardly walk. She was in pain all the time. She was nine months away from her death. Yet when we were with her there, she insisted on driving us to the clinic every day for her treatment. She couldn't walk without help, but she could drive, and it gave her a way of staying in life.

Also, don't make judgments about what people can and cannot do. Ask them. Just because a person is paralyzed from the waist down doesn't mean he or she can't think. Just because a person is sick doesn't mean he or she can't paint or write or play cards or think. Let people contribute whatever they can for as long as they can.

Don't . . .

Be Late

When you're taking care of someone who is seriously ill, being late will be more than an annoyance. Once when someone was late taking Susan to a hospital for admittance, the hospital was just about to give away the bed when we got there. If you're late, your friend may miss seeing a doctor. If you're late to relieve another group member, that person may miss an important appointment—or worse, may lose trust in you as a valuable member of the team.

If you find yourself consistently late in your group duties, especially if you've always been a prompt, on-time kind of person, you may want to examine your feelings to see if you're unconsciously avoiding dealing with illness and hospitals. Perhaps you should consider taking on less time-sensitive tasks for the group.

To people with a serious illness, time is very precious. They may realize how little of it they have left. They may even have been told they have five years or two years or less to live. To try to understand how they feel, ask yourself what you would do (make a list) if the doctor told you that you had only one year to live. Repeat the exercise, pretending it's only six months.

Do . . .

Forget About Being a Caregiver for a While and Give to Yourself

- Buy some fragrant bath gel and take a long shower or bath.
- Get together with some friends you haven't seen in a while and have a good laugh.
- Read that new novel you haven't had time to start.
- Go to a double feature and have popcorn, candy, and a soda.
- Have both a manicure and a pedicure—and go for the hot coral polish this time.
- Try some new exotic flavor of ice cream and . . . have a double dip.
- Go fishing.
- Play some peaceful music or meditate.
- Visit an art gallery, museum, or photo exhibit and get a new perspective on the world.
- Take your dog for a run in the park.
- Make a picnic lunch and go for a drive in the country.
- Plant some flowers, pick some flowers, arrange some flowers, buy some flowers.
- Get a massage.
- Go shopping.

Don't . . .

Buy into a Guilt Trip

It's not your fault that people get sick and you're healthy, yet they may unconsciously make you feel guilty for being able to do and have what they no longer can.

They may say things like "Well, how would you know what I'm going through? Nothing bad has ever happened to you!" Don't let them make you feel guilty for having been fortunate enough not to have had a tragic life. Every life has tragedies and loss, disappointments and pain, and physical illness isn't the only way human beings suffer.

Do . . .

Know the Difference Between Curing and Healing

In his book *Healing into Life and Death*, Steven Levine makes the point that a person's spirit may be healed and his body may still die.

There are many kinds of healing, and curing the body is only one of them. One person's lifelong anger may be healed. Another person may discover his or her creativity a few months before death.

Someone else may heal the rift in a close personal relationship, or say the "I love you" that had been unspoken for years. Another may get in touch with healthy anger.

Some people with caregiver groups will get better. Others will not. But in some way, there will be a healing. Leave room for the spiritual, emotional, and mental healing and acknowledge yourself for having had a part in it. Also acknowledge the patient and let your friend know that you don't think it's a failure to not beat disease. No matter what happens to the body, there may be a remarkable healing of the spirit.

Don't . . .

Assume Someone Can't Hear or Understand You

It is never a good idea to talk negatively or insensitively about sick people, assuming they are too sick, too old, or too medicated to hear you.

People who have had severe strokes have been able to recognize and respond to their loved ones. The elderly, who often seem confused, have moments of total clarity. Even people in comas have shown amazing responses.

Why take a careless chance of hurting someone's feelings or taking away a person's dignity or hope? Don't assume anything. Respect the person until the last moment.

Don't . . .

Try to Make Changes for the Elderly Without Their Approval or Support

If your group is helping out an elderly person, never attempt to make changes without their approval or support; you will only be creating a bigger problem. Older folks are less likely to feel open to major changes in their routines or their surroundings, especially if they are ill or losing their independence. They may think you are taking over their home or life and become fearful or angry. Take things slowly and give them time to consider your suggestions. Take baby steps. You need to gain their trust. The only time to really take a stand for change is when it is a health or safety issue.

Do . . .

Learn How to Say No as Well as Yes

Isn't it always the truth that the minute you say a quick yes to some commitment you really don't want to make, you feel angry, frustrated, and victimized?

As part of a caregiver group, you need to take responsibility for your decisions. As Dr. Miller often told us, "If they can't trust your no, they can't trust your yes." So the next time you are asked to do something:

- Think for a minute.
- Get all of the details of what is needed.
- Stop. Listen to yourself. How do you really feel about doing what you have been asked to do?
- If you feel you can fully accept the request, say yes.
- If you're not sure how you feel about it, ask for some time to think it over— and get back to the person within a specific amount of time.
- If you feel sure you don't want to do something, say no.
- Offer to do something else or to do the job at another time.

- You might also suggest someone else who might be able to do it or an alternative way of doing it.

The group doesn't want you to do the things you're afraid of or not good at. The group doesn't want you to be resentful or feel you're doing too much. The group needs you to say no as well as yes, and so does the person you are helping.

Do . . .

Break the Problem Up Into Little Pieces

- What *is* the problem? Listen to what is bothering your friend or fellow group member. Listen to what's not being said directly. What needs have to be met?
- Ask questions. Find out as much as possible about the situation so you can evaluate it effectively.
- Figure out all the possible options. Write them down. Consider the pros and cons of each one.
- Decide which one seems the best for the situation and act on it.
- Be prepared to discard it if it doesn't work, fit, or feel right, and try another option.
- Don't give up!

Do . . .

Encourage Your Friend to Join Support Groups

No one can truly understand the fears and pain of someone with a serious illness better than another person in the same shoes.

Do encourage your friend to join a support group and benefit from the weekly release of expressing feelings to other people with the same illness and to receive back their support. Knowing that others are going through similar journeys may help your friend feel less isolated and alone. Many studies have been made that point to the fact that this kind of support might even extend people's lives.

Call your local hospital, check with your friend's doctor, and contact support groups in your area that deal with your friend's specific illness.

Susan joined her local Cancer Care group and bonded with several women. They kept in touch long after Susan became too ill to continue to attend group meetings. One of them was Francine, whom we mention in the beginning of the book. Because of their talks and friendship, Francine had the courage to ask us to form her caregiver group.

Do . . .

Find Ways to Keep Your Friend Connected to Their Other Social Groups

A sense of isolation can be one of the most difficult feelings to handle for patients who have always led active, busy lives. Brainstorm possible ways to keep your friend connected with his or her past social groups

Most of Rick's men friends in Santa Fe came from a group he was part of called New Warriors. Though he tried to stay connected, it became impossible for him over time as his illness left him too weak to travel. At one point the entire group agreed to hold a meeting at Rick's house so he could participate. This turned out to be a very meaningful meeting for Rick and probably for his fellow members as well. Later three or four of them continued to hold small support group meetings at his home on a steady basis so Rick could still feel a connection to the whole group.

CHAPTER TWENTY-THREE

The Second Meeting: Ten Signals That It's Time to Have One

There came a point in the life of Susan's Funny Family when we needed desperately to have a meeting that did not include Susan. It was a time when even the most patient members were losing patience, even the most optimistic members were depressed, everyone was crying a lot, and most of us felt that we couldn't talk about our feelings in front of Susan. Susan had reached a turning point in her battle with cancer and we were at the breaking point.

We were all having a difficult time but none of us knew that everyone else was feeling the same way. Eventually we realized that we needed to share our feelings and adjust our systems. It wasn't really about Susan anymore. It was about us. If you recognize any one of the following ten signals, it is probably time for you to have your second meeting. Anyone can call this meeting, and if you do, you will see that everyone will be more than happy to attend.

The Ten Signals

1. There Has Been a Dramatic or Subtle Change in Your Sick Friend

Your friend's moods may swing radically from sweeping, dramatic abstractions ("Why did this happen to me? No one loves me!") to overly detailed, beat-by-beat descriptions of every medical procedure and trauma. They may be totally self-absorbed and unaware of anything but their own feelings. They may say they wish they were dead. They may be angry and totally unreasonable.

On the other hand, the changes may be very subtle but still disturbing. It might merely be that they don't walk around their apartment or home anymore but stay in one place. They've lost interest in the news, sports, music, or their favorite pastime. They can't spend the night alone anymore. They may be fully present one moment, then drift away and seem to be somewhere else in another dimension.

It may be that their physical environment has subtly changed. A hospital bed has been brought in. A part-time nurse is there one day when you arrive. There are many signs that things have somehow changed. If you're working with the person or are there all the time, you may miss the subtle signs.

2. Someone Who Isn't in the Group and Hasn't Been There in Months Arrives and Is Shocked

The changes in your friend and his or her environment are so incremental and subtle that sometimes it takes an objective person to alert you to them. Pay attention if an old friend arrives and says, "My God! She looks so different!" Or "When did these bars go up in the bathroom? When did he start needing a wheelchair? What happened? Why is there a nurse's aide sitting in the corner?" You haven't registered this consciously because it's been happening bit by bit over a long time, but somewhere in your gut you *have* registered it, and the turning point is very upsetting. It's time for a second meeting.

3. One Way or Another, Everyone Is Going Crazy

Or, if they're not going crazy, they're frayed at the edges. Whereas they were able to do one more thing, stretch a little further, or be flexible six months ago, people aren't anymore. They may assume they're worn out because it's been a long time, but it may be that these subtle changes are going on and they haven't registered them. So they're anxious and fearful but don't quite know why.

4. The Person Who Is Ill Is Changing

The environment of the person who is ill is changing. At the same time, more is being demanded by the sickness. So the personality of the person who is sick is responding to what's going on. They are getting more irritable, more agitated, more concerned about themselves. They remember that not that long ago they said things like "I'm never going to be in a hospital bed. I'm never going to go for chemotherapy! You're never going to see me in dialysis!" Now they remember those vows and know (inside) that step by step they've changed. First it was the cane, then the walker, then the grip bars in the bathroom, then the nurse who comes in twice a week, now the hospital bed in the living room.

5. The Person Who Is Ill Has Been Irritable with Everybody but Everyone in the Group Thinks It's Just Them

At this stage, it's not unusual for members of the group to assume that they've done something wrong. You haven't had a lot of group meetings, so people may not have shared their stories and feelings. You may feel you're the only one getting irritated and angry and that it's somehow not right to gossip about or bad-mouth your sick friend. This is a very heavy burden to carry alone.

6. The Person Who Is Ill Is Telling Everyone That Everybody Else in the Group Is Incompetent

No matter how much everybody does, it's not enough, it's not right, it's not good enough, fast enough, thorough enough.

7. The Group Is Dwindling (You're Losing People)

In reality, the person who is ill has been irritable with everybody, everybody is feeling something has changed, and everybody wants to run away. Suddenly, the captains can't find enough people to fill the schedule for the week. Someone drops out of the group due to a big project at work, someone else simply can't be reached.

8. Systems Are Breaking Down

No one can remember whose turn it is to be captain. No one is volunteering for any jobs. Someone loses the oncologist's phone number at a critical time. What was working perfectly before seems to be in total disarray.

9. The Biological Family Is Coming More Often

If your caregiver "family" has been taking almost total care of your sick friend, it may be very hard to step aside when a real sister or cousin or mother shows up and wants to be the main caregiver. You may even resent the appearance of a long-lost husband or daughter. These feelings are real and another indication that you need to talk about them.

10. Everyone in the Group Is Closer Than Ever, and Yet Everyone Feels Alone

You've had lunch together, done difficult jobs together, dried each other's tears, shared secrets, and had deep conversations about the meaning of it all. You've been operating like a close-knit family, yet suddenly, for no reason you can think of, you feel totally alone.

It's time to have a second meeting.

CHAPTER TWENTY-FOUR

The Second Meeting: The Agenda

Support and Acknowledgment

Dr. Miller started our second meeting by passing out blue ribbons to each of us and saying: "I am in awe of the job you have all been doing. I acknowledge all your hard work, your going beyond the call of duty, your compassion, and your dedication. Bravo. Congratulations."

We were stunned. As far as we knew, things were falling apart, Susan was miserable, we were failing. We were also very moved by her simple yet profound gesture. It had been a long time since we had acknowledged each other or ourselves. It had been a long time since we had gotten together and shared as the "family" we had become.

Yet this meeting was as important as our very first meeting. Your second meeting is one the person who is ill will not attend. Tell him or her you're having a meeting to reorganize. Here, there are no exercises, no forms. The keynote is sharing and acknowledgment.

Set it up to be warm and nurturing. Have a meal together. Have everyone cook a favorite dish and bring it. Have everyone bring a thank-you card. Put them all in a bowl and have everyone pick one. Award each other for all the work and effort. Give each other the acknowledgment you may no longer be getting from the patient, who has become more and more preoccupied with his or her own situation.

Remember, because systems are failing, the patient is failing, and energy is failing, it's easy for people to feel that *they're* failing, that they're doing something wrong. You have to be there for each other to say "Don't panic, this is a natural stage."

Share with each other where you are. Just spill it out. Say everything. There's no right or wrong. Share what you're all worried about, concerned about, what you're disappointed in, what you're angry about, even if it seems inappropriate. Here's an honest quote from our second meeting:

> I remember we had a meeting without Susan and she was pissed to be left out. Different women began to complain about Susan . . . about her impatience, her attitude. They expressed their aggravation and anger toward her. A few were burnt out. I was brought up to always try to please, to make everyone appreciate me and like me and never to show these kinds of "hostile" feelings, or to suffer endless guilt if I ever allowed even a thought in that direction. A martyr is a saint and we should all strive for sainthood. Here these women were talking about what a royal pain Susan could be and I was totally shocked! And relieved! How free to really feel your real feelings and not hate yourself or jump to change yourself or deny yourself . . . just let it out and there it is and it doesn't mean I don't love Susan. It was definitely a new world for me (L.R.)

Setting Affairs in Order

If your friend is facing death, it may be that everyone in the group is increasingly anxious as to whether that person's affairs are in order. Is there a will? Does anyone have access to the bank account? Have arrangements for a funeral or burial been made? Who will take care of the kids, the businesses, the pets? By now, many of these things have probably been taken care of, but if you or your sick friend have avoided these issues, now is the time to address them. Don't panic. You probably have more information than you think. You may at this point want to appoint someone to deal with these issues. For help on this, refer to chapter 20, "Getting Their Affairs in Order."

Adjusting Systems

Often, systems break down at about the same time the patient has taken a turn for the worse. Jobs aren't getting filled. Schedules are getting harder to keep. People aren't communicating. The captain's schedule hasn't been updated in two months. One caregiver group we know of even complained about being split into the "talkers" and the "doers."

Because you're all so frayed, it may seem like a huge job to get your group back on track. But think back to your first meeting and initial planning sessions. Put those systems back into play, perhaps with some modifications, and once again your group will function like a well-oiled machine. You'll come up with the answers quickly and easily. Remember, you already know how the systems work, you know each others' skills, and you know what's possible and what's not.

Say to the group, "What's working? What's not working?" Maybe you need more people on weekends. Maybe people are complaining about too many e-mails. If friends who've heard about your group have offered to help, now's the time to call on them. Expand your free-floaters. Prepare for more real family involvement. Adjust to the fact that the biological family may now need to be there more than you and that the nurse may need to be there all the time.

But more than anything else, listen to each other, share with each other, and acknowledge each other. Because now it isn't only about the sick person anymore. It's about you.

CHAPTER TWENTY-FIVE

Confronting Yourself

No matter how much you love your friend and how much you truly want to help, being with someone who is seriously ill can be very taxing emotionally. Not only is it upsetting to bear witness to a friend's pain and fear, but many of your sick friend's feelings can spill over onto you.

Do not be surprised if at times you find you are on an emotional roller coaster. This problem is made doubly difficult because, in fact, *you are there for your sick friend; he or she cannot be there for you.* All of your friend's time and energy must be spent in coping with a dramatically changed life. Although it is difficult to acknowledge in situations where one tends to the sick, the caregiver has needs also.

You may well experience the same range of emotions as the person you are taking care of. This may seem strange because, after all, you are not sick. But you are human.

We have found that no matter how inappropriate some of our feelings seemed to us at the time, in sharing them with one another we were able to feel natural and normal again. This is one of the greatest things you and your group can do for one another: to give permission and support to one another's feelings whether they seem selfish, uncaring, strange, or stupid. They are real, they are part of being a caregiver, and with acknowledgment and support, they pass. Only another caregiver can truly understand what you are feeling.

So as these feelings come up, share them with others in your group and know that no matter how inappropriate some of your feelings may seem, they are the natural and normal feelings of all caregivers.

You Feel Guilty for Being Healthy

You are working as hard as you can in your caregiver group. You fulfill all your responsibilities well, on time, and with pleasure. From time to time, you have even totally rearranged your own schedule to fulfill your obligations.

You'd give anything if your friend could be not sick. You haven't done anything wrong, anything bad, or anything irresponsible, but you feel guilty. It is not uncommon for caregivers to feel guilty for being healthy when the person they love is suffering.

> When I was helping my brother-in-law, I felt guilt, pressure, and maybe some resentments. The guilt was when I was not available, the pressure was when I didn't have the energy, the resentments when I thought some others in my family could be doing more. (T.M.)

It is not uncommon for caregivers to feel guilty for being able to do the things, eat the things, and enjoy the things that their loved one can no longer do, eat, enjoy, and accomplish. Sometimes, in their darkest moments, it is not uncommon for the sick person to wittingly or unwittingly provoke your guilt.

> Susan was very fond of saying to me, "Oh, you've led a charmed life. Nothing bad has ever happened to you. How would *you* know how I feel?" (T.P.)

The Results of Guilt

If you feel guilty enough, you may (unconsciously) neglect your own health, you may volunteer for more than you really want to do, you may drive yourself to exhaustion as a way of punishing yourself. So when guilt surfaces, remember that you're doing all you can and that no one has all the answers.

You're Angry at Your Friend for Getting Sick

Many people blame themselves when a loved one gets sick ("If I had only insisted he go to a specialist earlier" or "If I had only noticed something was wrong"). But it's equally common to blame the person with the disease. We say, "If he had only gone to the doctor earlier. If he had only changed his diet, given up smoking, begun that exercise program, been more sexually responsible." Usually the caregiver blames the sick person silently—and feels guilty about that, too.

In our blame, what we may really be doing is searching desperately to make sense of the illness. One reason we do this is because it is very hard for most of us to deal with the things we don't understand. Another is that we believe if we can pinpoint the cause of the illness, maybe we can keep it from happening to us. But even people who take good care of themselves get sick. The best people in the world get hurt. Young people die, children die, and there never seems to be a reason.

There is no answer why a forty-two-year-old woman who should be in the prime of her life is dying. Or why a child should die from cancer. It is important to remember that even strong, young men and women, even innocent children, even people who take very good care of themselves, get sick. So we have to confront the randomness, the unfairness of the universe. We have to deal with the reality that it could happen to us.

Sometimes, you will be angry for other reasons. Maybe you're angry because not only are you giving up so much to take care of your friend, but he or she doesn't seem to appreciate it. Maybe you're angry because you're losing someone who has always been there for you. Maybe losing this person will leave an incredible gap in your life. Maybe your own kids have just gotten out of the house, you're finally free to pursue a hobby or interest, and now you have to take care of an ailing friend.

Sometimes the anger is simply that we feel the human rage at the fact that we all must die. Frequently, it is only in caring for critically ill people that we come into contact with this rage. When we are experiencing it, painful as it is, we are also experiencing our profound connection to one another.

Whatever the cause of your anger, don't deny it, minimize it, or ignore it. Try to have compassion for yourself, respect it, find a healthy way to express it, and know that all caregivers feel it at one time or another.

You're Convinced You're Sick Yourself

It is a very common thing for people in their first year of medical school to imagine they have all kinds of illnesses. The same is true for caregivers. You may see a pimple and imagine you have cancer, or lose weight and be certain you're HIV positive. You may run to doctors all the time for mammograms, blood tests, checkups, only to be told over and over that nothing is wrong. Or you may avoid going to the doctor entirely, paralyzed with fear. Again, just know that this happens to many caregivers, and if it's acknowledged and understood, it passes in time.

The Pain You Didn't Know Was There

As the person who is ill confronts the pain of loss, the pain of limitations, the pain of its being too late, you may feel old wounds come to the surface . . . a painful incident from childhood, an abortion never fully dealt with, an accident you feel you caused. If you've buried a lot of painful memories, have never come to terms with your own losses and failures, this can be quite intense. It might not even make sense. They may be crying about the loss of an arm and you may suddenly feel the pain of a totally unrelated personal loss.

Getting Help Yourself

To deal with your own feelings, you may need to lean on another member of the group, a co-worker, a friend, a husband. You may need to see a therapist. Most of all, you may need to rely on someone else to tell you how you're doing. When you're a caregiver you may not see how exhausted you are. You may "not be yourself" and not know it. Trust other group members. They know what you're going through. When they tell you you need a break, take it. If your boss says your work is not up to par, listen. Remember, if you don't get the help you need, you can't help your friend.

The Questions You Never Asked

At some point, you may find it hard to make small talk with someone who is seriously ill. The patient will be shockingly frank, probing, and may be asking some very tough questions. Is my life fulfilling? Am I doing what I wanted to do? Why don't I have someone to love? Do I like my life? One of the most painful things sick people may confront is the time they wasted, the things they didn't do . . . that now they may never do. Did I give up my dreams? Is time running out for me? What does it all mean?

Susan asked herself many tough questions. Why did she work twelve hours a day? Why didn't she do something more creative or satisfying? What was she going to do now that she had to quit her job? Since many of us were women with careers, these issues made us ask the same questions. When she began to raise spiritual issues and ask questions about what happens after death, we asked them too. When, despite her illness, she questioned her relationships, we began to look at our own.

As the person who is ill confronts these overwhelming feelings, you will be forced to confront your own. As your friend wrestles with issues of life and death, you will wrestle with them too, and as your friend searches for the meaning of his or her life, you will search for the meaning of yours.

Even practical questions may plug you in. As they leave their job and begin to rely on disability insurance, or they try to pay their medical bills without it, you may suddenly realize you don't have any. As they make out or change their will, you may think about your own. As they deal with questions of Living Wills, cremations or burials, and funeral arrangements, you may realize you haven't dealt with these issues.

So in addition to confronting some overwhelming emotions, you may face a more subtle kind of inner confrontation as you ask those questions about your own life. This is perhaps the most difficult part of caregiving, and yet it is the part that can give you back the most.

At one point during the time I was taking care of my friend, everything began to plug me in. I watched how brave Susan was, the chances she was taking. Here she was with a terminal illness and she was taking workshops, writing a screenplay, trying to do freelance work at home. She was really living and I felt like my life was on hold. I began to realize I too was going to die one day and I'd better get on with it while I had the chance. (C.R.P.)

Try to see all this as an opportunity for you to grow, to change your life for the better, and to prepare for the future. Talk about your feelings as they arise. Share with other members of the group. Remember, the only emotions that will truly damage you or them are the ones you don't acknowledge.

Don't Pretend It Isn't Hard

Caregiving may be one of the most demanding things you will ever do. Acknowledge yourself and let other people in the group acknowledge you. Give yourself a treat after a tough assignment. Take a relaxing shower or a hot bath. Water seems to actually wash away the vibrations of illness, to renew you, and to restore you to yourself.

Forgive Yourself

Forgive yourself for not having all the answers, for not being able to cure illness or ease pain. Forgive yourself for not being perfect. No one knows how to do this perfectly. No one has all the answers. Own your own goodness and acknowledge yourself for doing whatever you can do.

How Much Giving Is Enough?

No one can tell you how much to do or what is enough. Dr. Miller once said to us, "Do whatever you need to do so that when Susan is gone you will feel complete and not have any regrets."

CHAPTER TWENTY-SIX

Changes

No matter how much you're committed to the group, you may have to make some individual changes to be an effective caregiver family member. These changes won't be the same for everyone.

1. You may need to limit your commitments while you're an active part of a caregiver group, especially if you're the type of person who always takes on too much. Assume that if the total amount of stress points you can handle is ten, you've already used up at least four. See what you can take out of your schedule. If you've always wanted to take that extra course at night or run a marathon, this may not be the time.

2. You may need to put energy back into your own life, especially if you're the type of person who frequently ignores her own needs. Sign up for that art or photography class. Get your own hopes and dreams back on track again. Start doing yoga at the health club again. Fix up your workshop and get that long-forgotten project into the works.

    Sheila notes: "While part of the group, I started painting again. Not only was it creatively satisfying, but the quality and quantity of work that poured out of me at this time was astounding. Within two and a half years, I had put together a one-woman show."

3. You may need to spend extra time planning, especially if you tend to do things on the spur of the moment. Leave space for the fact that the transition from your normal life to your role as caregiver requires a psychological shift as well as perhaps a physical one. You may not be able to go from the gym to a meet-

ing to a radiation appointment without some assimilation time in between. Take extra time to plan your schedule, thinking through your commitments, logistics, and meetings. If logistics and planning are not your long suit, ask another member of the group to help you.

Also, reduce the unknowns in the rest of your life so you have space for the crises in your sick friend's life. Leave room for the unexpected.

4. You may need to let go of schedules and certainty, especially if you tend to cling to structure. As part of a group, you may be asked to react or respond quickly. Be willing to trust your instincts and roll with the punches.

5. You may need to be honest at work, especially if you tend to bear everything alone. You may have to tell your boss, secretary, employees, and others that you are involved in a caregiver group. This is not as easy as it sounds. Most of us want to keep our work lives and our private lives separate—and with good reason. However, it could hurt you not to be honest. Inevitably, there will be times when you may be late, distracted, or not at top form. If people don't know the reason, many will assume you are being irresponsible, or that you're having personal problems, even drug or alcohol problems, or that you simply don't care. If you do share what you're doing, you may be surprised to find how supportive people really are when they find out that what you're doing is for somebody else.

Changes You Should Not Make in Your Own Life

1. You cannot give up the things that make you happy. Don't give up the things that give you pleasure or keep you going.

Cappy cites an important example: "My hobby was ballroom dancing, and at the beginning Susan loved to hear about my latest steps, see my latest ball gowns, and live vicariously through me. As she got sicker and began to lose more and more mobility, I began to feel guilty dancing while my friend was walking with a cane. But I realized that dancing was what kept me going, kept me healthy, and that the energy of the dance studio renewed me. It wasn't necessary to give it up, just to stop sharing it with Susan."

2. Do not try to do caretaking twenty-four hours a day. Sickness has a palpable, real energy. It drains you. It takes incredible energy. It's exhausting to be around. No one can do it twenty-four hours a day.

3. Don't isolate yourself from your "healthy" friends. You need to laugh, to relax, to be frivolous, to have fun even if someone very close to you can't.

CHAPTER TWENTY-SEVEN

The Closing Meeting: Why You Need to Have One

At some point, your Share The Care group will need to come together and say good-bye in a final closing meeting. This will happen when the need for the group has ended. If your friend has recovered from his or her illness or has gotten past a crisis (for example, a bone-marrow transplant or a serious operation) and is no longer in need of you, getting closure is important and a celebration may be in order. If your friend has died, a closing meeting is still important, perhaps more so. Even if your friend has decided to go and live with his mother in another state or in a climate that is better for his health and has moved away, you still need a closing meeting.

There are two important reasons to come together at this time. One is that even though the key motivation for forming the group is no longer there, the many important and nurturing relationships that have formed in the course of the group's operation are still there and need to be acknowledged.

The other is that all of you have been living "on alert" for a long time, and you must accept that it is over so that your mind and body can truly let go and move on. You no longer have to be a captain, cook dinner on Thursday nights, or drive your friend to a weekly chemotherapy appointment.

The Importance of Closure

There are important reasons for the ritual of closure. Whether it's a PTA meeting, a business partnership or corporation, a graduation ceremony, or a retirement party, such rituals are more than just an acknowledgment of individuals. They are an acknowledgment of individuals in their relationships to teammates, business colleagues, classmates—to other people.

In coming together as a caregiver family, you have formed a group that is greater than any of its individual pieces, a group that has persevered through darkness and pain and brought beauty and love to someone in need and to each other. It was a group that did things most people wouldn't have believed possible. Now, everyone needs to be acknowledged for the part they played in this.

CHAPTER TWENTY-EIGHT

The Closing Meeting: The Agenda

In order for your final Share The Care meeting to really be of value to each and every member, there are some guidelines you will want to follow.

When to Have the Meeting

The time to have the meeting will be approximately one month after the need for the group has ended. Arrange to have it at someone's home or some other place that will allow for your sharing and affirming to be private. Only those people who were part of the group should attend. It is also extremely important to make sure everyone involved is able to attend. You may find some of your members are still in pain (if your friend has died) and will need extra encouragement to attend. But the valuable affirmation and acknowledgments of this meeting are so rewarding that every single one of you should be there to receive them.

A Gift for Everyone

You, as group members, have given of yourselves for so long. It is now time to receive a small, symbolic gift for your efforts, love, and hard work. We would suggest that each member bring a small, inexpensive gift. It should be beautifully wrapped and somehow be a remembrance of this time together as caregivers. All the gifts should be placed in the center of the table so everyone can choose one.

Make the receiving of the gifts an event. Let each person open a gift and enjoy a moment in the spotlight. You may be touched by the ingenuity, thought, meaning, and love that went into the choosing of these token gifts.

Share the Best and the Worst of Times

After you have opened the gifts you may want to casually tell some stories about being in the group. Some will be funny, some will be sad, but all will be meaningful and will remind everyone of what an incredible job they have all done.

What may also come up are feelings people have about what they consider to be the mistakes they made. "If only I had been there that day, she wouldn't have fallen . . ." Or "If only I had paid closer attention to how he was feeling I could have alerted the doctor sooner." When people share such feelings they will elicit responses from their fellow group members. "No, she would have fallen anyway; those tiles were always wet and slippery after the rain. It was just one of those things." Or "You're not a medical professional; you did the best you could do." This exchange is very valuable. In sharing, some members will be receiving important words of forgiveness and understanding from others who have shared the caregiving experience.

Saying Good-bye for Now

When Susan died, we had our closing meeting and said good-bye, but it wasn't for long. To this day, many of the members of Susan's Share The Care group who started out as complete strangers have stayed in touch, and some have become fast friends. As time goes on, we realize that in some way we will always remain "Susan's Funny Family."

PART 5

Beyond the Group: Changed Lives

CHAPTER TWENTY-NINE

Personal Meaning

When someone is confronted with a life-threatening illness, many questions come to the surface and demand answers. "What is the meaning of my life?" "What have I done to make a difference?" "What will I leave of lasting value?" "Who will remember me?"

When Susan began asking those questions, we began asking them as well, and we realized it was important to answer them whether we were faced with serious illness or not. Personal meaning took many forms for us.

Coming through for Susan enabled many of us to come through for other people in our lives . . . our lovers, our friends, our spouses, our parents and children, and perhaps most important, ourselves. Going the extra step for her made us realize we could go the extra distance for ourselves. Dealing with her problems put our own problems in a different perspective. We stopped complaining about the small stuff. In one way, we began to lighten up about ourselves, to stop taking ourselves so seriously. In another, we began to take ourselves more seriously, as we realized we could be counted on.

As we watch the courage of people faced with death, we begin to find the courage to live a more authentic life. We stop procrastinating. We stop blaming our troubles on other people. We begin to do the things we've always wanted to do. Perhaps most important of all, we begin to live not in the future, not in a dream, not in denial, but in the moment. When we do, we see how rich each moment is, how full each day, how precious the little things.

Here are some of the ways in which people who participated in Share The Care families describe the personal meaning they found in the experience:

You Feel Like You're Living a Richer, More Authentic Life

I look at life differently now. I spend more time with positive influences, try to enjoy life more, and don't get as upset with things that in the past would have greatly upset me. Everyone, once in their life, should have the opportunity to experience people working together to help other people. There's no better fulfillment in life than to know that maybe you made one hour, one day, or more a little brighter for someone. (A.R.)

I got to really know Susan and get a firsthand lesson in courage and great humor in the midst of trauma, distress, and pain. As for the group, I felt women sharing real respect for each other, true sensitivity, and instant warm camaraderie. (C.R.P.)

The group was about life and death, fear and caring, courage and setbacks, human spirit and frustration, hope and acceptance and fate. It was about having little control, facing that, making a moment count, and finding ways of endlessly coping under the worst possible conditions. (T.K.)

I feel so much older now. "Life" is so much more serious to me now. (S.V.)

You Feel You Are Able to Accept More Help

I always believed that whatever had to be done should be done by me. That was my duty in life, to "do the deed," "be responsible," "fix every situation," "soothe every person." And if I did not respond and do whatever needed doing, that "it wouldn't get done right." It's so controlling and so vain. And yet it never felt like vanity or arrogance—it felt like helpfulness—like I had no other choice. But these women [in the group] were as good as—or better than—me, smarter than me, more imaginative and creative than me, more qualified and capable than me. Maybe better for Susan than me! It was a humbling realization. And it took away the weight and burden I carried. I could totally trust that they were there for Susan and that I didn't really need to do it all. And I didn't need to feel *guilty*—I could be grateful! (K.T.)

Getting closer with Susan as I spent more time with her was very rewarding. This was because I was getting a different kind of attention from her than I had ever experienced. I found that as I gave more to Susan, she gave more back to me. When my dad was dying, I spent time talking to Susan. She was more compassionate toward me and my pain than she had ever been. (J.J.)

Lois, as I've said, could not cry and would not ask for anything. But that changed—to have her call me to come over and calm her down when the steroids made her wild. I told her how much I learned through her as she struggled to conquer her illness—she told me how much she learned from me and how calming an influence I was for her—we shared a great deal. (M.K.)

You Feel You Are Able to Connect in a Deeper Way

No other group I had been in had a shared goal. We were there primarily to get Susan through this battle . . . anything else that occurred did so secondarily. In other groups (business and therapy) I've never experienced this depth of feelings. (L.T.)

It was most rewarding helping someone in need. Maybe I couldn't stop the cancer, but I could spend time with Lois and make her feel like the human being she is—not just someone riddled with cancer and pumped up with drugs. I'm happy I was able to make her life easier in the end. (S.S.)

It was in my head that Dr. Miller kind of "stirred" us together years ago and we "formed." "We" became something different, separate—an energy? a force? Something that has its own life, apart from all of us. Like a "force" that gets passed, like a mantle, to each new group . . . and gets "worn" by each new Share The Care family. (A.R.)

Being in the group I got a feeling of bonding and participation I never expected. We were able to speak to each other and boost each other in a very personal way, even though I never met most of the other members before. (W.F.)

Family is not always defined by blood or marriage, but more often by love and commitment to each other. (B.B.)

You Learn to Go the Distance

I discovered that I am very strong . . . that I have emotional limits where I need to recharge . . . that I am not afraid of death, rather the tragedy of how poorly we can lead our lives . . . that after all these years we have come so short a distance with cancer. (W.G.)

I discovered that I was able to function under this extreme emotional distress. (L.N.)

I can help when it counts, and that is a very rewarding feeling. (C.L.)

I learned that I am more compassionate and understanding than I think I am. My patience and tolerance level were tested many times, but I've learned to use my energy in helpful ways. (T.M.)

You Feel Good About Yourself and What You Are Doing

My involvement was a continuing source of interest and awe to my family and friends. The concept and cohesive functioning of the group drew frequent [comments of] "How terrific," "It's wonderful!" and "You women are fabulous." Compliments and endless questions of concern, curiosity, and praise, praise, praise. (F.S.)

I was familar with cancer and death from a professional, clinical point of view. But here was Susan, someone I knew and liked and grew fonder of as time went on. She was close to my age and I guess I identified with her. I did not realize it at the time but my membership in the [group] was to be part of a preparation for the future for me. It prepared me for my own aunt's illness and death this year. Until Susan (and one other friend who died in 1985), dealing with sickness and death was just part of the job. Through these experiences, especially Susan's, I gained a lot of insight, suffered a lot of pain and loss, and became, I believe, a better nurse and person as a result. (A.L.)

You know that the more you give, the more you will like yourself. There is such a feeling of well-being, of satisfaction, of pride in giving to someone else that you become more sure of yourself, more proud of yourself. A self-esteem that comes from this self-respect. (E.B.)

You Conquer Your Deepest Fears

One way or the other you will all survive the experience, and many more good things will come out of it than you could have imagined in your wildest dreams. It's hard to see that in the beginning. In the beginning there's just "fear"—then . . . everyone gets to work. Each member brings their own resources to the situation—each person learns to reach deep inside and bring something of unique value to the situation, a sense of humor, comfort, support, a warm touch, a phone call, a dinner that takes the edge off of the day. (J.W.)

Being in the group was an experience I will never forget! Someone I cared for had died. But her death was a lesson. I saw the strength of the human instinct to survive, and then to realize that there would be no survival. My fear of death is still with me but I think of Susan and the fear lessens. I also met the most wonderful group of women. The power of women's feelings, emotions, realness, and commitment made me proud of what we accomplished. (T.P.)

I learned "the facts of life"—that we all will die. Somehow it isn't as frightening as it was. And that if we ask for help, it's there. And though we may feel alone, if we have the courage to let others in, others will be there. (R.A.)

CHAPTER THIRTY

The Healing Journey

What we've seen in one caregiver family after another is that whether the person who is ill gets well or dies, a profound healing seems to take place. It's a unique kind of healing . . . the kind that comes from having the combined strength of a group around you.

Everyone has the ability to heal, but the form of healing is different for each of us. Some of us heal with our hands, some with our laughter, some with our stories, some with our faith. We heal with the funny get well card, the homemade lasagna, the lighting of a candle. We heal by having the courage to tell the truth. We heal others out of the things we've come to terms with in our own life—our own pain, our own disappointments, our own illnesses.

When a person has a Share The Care family, that person has the benefit of a hundred kinds of healing coming toward him or her all at once, like many colored rays of light. The healing power of each individual becomes stronger, magnified, as it merges with the group's.

Every group finds unique ways to heal the person in its care, and every person who has been cared for by a group has a unique story. But something else seems to happen in Share The Care groups. The kindnesses flowing toward the person who is ill spill out and touch the other members, and ultimately, the healers heal each other.

Philip's Story

Philip, an associate professor of literature at Lake Forest College, suffered from ALS and had a group of forty men, women, and teens known as FOPAK (Friends Of Phil And Kathryn—his wife). Philip came across Share The Care in 1998, after battling his illness for three years, and it was he who suggested to friends it might be the best way to help him.

While his body was becoming weaker he authored a beautiful book called *Learning to Fall: The Blessings of an Imperfect Life.** It is filled with wisdom, humor, and amazing observations. This is his incredible legacy. His wife, Kathryn, describes the journey:

> Phil wrote on his own for the good part of the ten years. Later he wrote daily on the computer, using voice recognition hardware. As his ALS progressed and he had trouble with the voice recognition system, he switched to another system that operated using a light-sensitive dot attached to his glasses that pointed to letters on the screen. It was very slow and frustrating for Phil. That frustration and physical exhaustion led him to ask others to type for him. The book *Learning to Fall* was written completely on his own. It took his whole focus and also provided his inspiration to keep living.

> The letters, phone calls, and invitations to speak that came after self-publishing *Learning to Fall* were what gave him the fuel to keep trying to live. He experienced that his work touched people's lives and made a difference. The ALS was terrible, but he had his brain, intelligence, sense of humor, drive, and voice to put his experience into words, and that was a great gift to him as well as to all who knew him in person and through the writing. He was my hero in his commitment to live life fully and to find pleasure in each day.

Linda's Story

Linda's Share The Care Group in Wisconsin consisted of forty-two men, woman, teens, and children. Leukemia took Linda's life after one short

---

* See Helpful Books, page 323.

year. Her group dedicated a memorial bench by Lost Lake at Saint Benedict Center in her memory. Her daughter Aymee told us how the group continues to heal by honoring Linda's memory yearly.

A Share The Care Team is a lifelong gift, not only for the recipient, but for the family of the person in need. We now meet as a group each year on the anniversary of Linda's death to celebrate her life. These are truly amazing people.

Francine's Story

Here is what Francine had to say about her Share The Care group, a group that has been taking care of her for more than three years, a group that raised over $30,000 to pay for her medical treatments.

Without my group, I would have been paralyzed. I was constantly going to doctors. I had no money and no insurance. I had this tremendous fear: How am I going to pay for my Medicare supplement? How am I going to pay for my bone marrow transplant? They were brilliant. They went so far beyond the call of duty. I said I needed money, and bing, bang, boom, there it was!

It was an amazing fund-raising effort. First, they went to the local paper and the editor sent a reporter to interview me. They put my picture on the front page and let people know there was going to be a fund-raiser. They put mayonnaise jars in local stores with my picture on them. I was getting money from people all over Brooklyn. Then they rented a place and did an auction. A singing group called the Classics sang pro bono. One member's father, who was an artist, donated one of his paintings. An interior decorator member donated picture frames. My ex-boss donated a day's temp service. My brother Peter donated a time share "anywhere in the world"! And my older brother donated clothes from his boutique. My ex-fiancé (who had won the Lotto) sent $5,000. Another friend offered a day of free housecleaning. The donations just kept coming. My group raised over $15,000. Then, while I was in the hospital, they threw a

"Valentine's Day Gala," a dance with a band, and raised several thousand more. They had a white elephant sale.

At my fund-raiser, I tried to thank them, and I remember my words: "I can now dispute the cliché that blood is thicker than water. I have an extended family that is my family. You are absolutely incredible. I want you all to know that you are my source of strength, my courage. You comfort me, you cry with me, you laugh with me. You have been my medicine. I love you from the bottom of my heart."

Carol's Story

Carol's Share The Care group came together overnight and has just celebrated a three-year anniversary. It began with more than twenty women and then expanded to include the husbands of several of the women and other male friends. Although they are a group of professional women and men with big responsibilities, they continue to carve a niche out of their busy lives for Carol. This is what Carol had to say about her support group:

> My support group has become the highway my life travels on. I dare not think about what my life would be without their support. Giving up is not an option they have given me nor one I have given myself. They saved my life and they continue to do so.

Lois's Story

Lois's Share The Care group had very little time with Lois because her cancer took her very quickly, but her group found strength together and expressed how moved they were by creating a quilt to honor Lois's life.

Though they intended it for her, it ended up being a healing gift for her family. The quilt was presented to Lois's parents at her memorial service. This is how Eileen, a member of Susan's group who attended Lois's service, described it in a letter:

> Two of Lois's close friends presented to her parents an extraordinary quilt "in memory of Lois, and so much like Lois . . . warm and comforting."

You would not believe the quilt . . . patches and squares made by each of her friends . . . every piece a message or a memorial to Lois.

- A patchwork heart
- A sky with sunshine and birds
- A big yellow flower
- Animals snuggling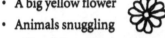
- A "beach" square—miniature sunglasses, seashells, and beach balls
- A caricature of Lois in her "body-building phase"
- Large and small and skinny and fat. Squares with people's names and loving remarks and . . . in the lower right corner, a rectangle that said:

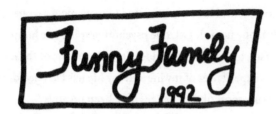

Some of you know that I've always felt silly calling us the "Funny Family"—it never came smoothly off my tongue, and I still rarely say it. It's hard to describe the "thunk" I felt in my stomach when I saw that patch.

Susan's Story

Perhaps the greatest example of a healing came to Susan herself. Though her body wasn't healed, her spirit was. She often said she lived more fully and more creatively in the last four years of her life than in all the others combined. Susan, who had always been a somewhat driven business-woman, not given to reflection or introspection, began to explore her creativity when she was moved to write about her "Funny Family." Someone told her about a storytelling course given by Spalding Gray at the Omega Institute. To get into the course, you had to write a one-page letter. Out of thousands of applicants, Susan was one of twelve people chosen. This was her letter.

SUSAN FARROW
67 West 80th Street
New York, N.Y. 10017

April 20, 1989

Omega Institute
Att: True Stories

It is now five years that I am living with this mysterious disease called cancer. Up to this point I have had three surgeries, forty-seven days of radiation, three bone scans, one MRI, one myelogram and at least one million blood tests. I have accumulated two oncologists, one surgeon, one orthopedist, one neurologist, one psychotherapist, one homeopathist and tons of nurses, technicians and aides. It has been one of the most terrifying, horrendous experiences of my life and my life has changed dramatically. Yet, to my surprise, most of the changes have been positive.

One of the most amazing things to come out of this was a group that became known as Susan's Funny Family. Sukie, my wonderful therapist, gathered together twelve of my closest friends to explain to them how they could help me survive my sixth tumor crisis.

They physically and emotionally took over my life. They handled the cooking, the shopping, the doctors, the hospital, the insurance forms, everything! Without their help and unsparing love, I would not have survived mentally, let alone physically.

This is my story that I told to another friend, Loudon Wainwright, a writer for *Life* magazine. He thought it was so inspiring that he encouraged me to get it down on paper.

And so it began. I borrowed a typewriter and quickly realized that this writing business was not so easy. Among other problems, the Funny Family Story just couldn't be appreciated out of the context of my whole experience with cancer. So I had to start from the beginning, from the very first lump!

Although writing my story has been very emotional for me, it has also been an enormous psychological healing process. And along with the help from Sukie, I have learned so much about what my life wasn't about, what people are really about and exactly what the quality of life could be. Loudon passed away before I had the courage to show him a draft of my story and somehow the impetus to get it done died too.

When I saw the workshop description, I couldn't believe it. I felt so inspired to pick up the story again, but I don't know quite how to do it. Little did I suspect that cancer would be the beginning of the end of the life I knew. I've learned so much and I do think some of what I've experienced might just help someone else, somehow.

I would very much like to get help in finishing my story and then see where it can go.

Sincerely yours,
Susan Farrow

Final Message from the Authors

From Cappy

When Susan and I were writing together, we skirted around the issue of her dying for months and months, using the screenplay as a way of fictionalizing reality, pretending that what was happening was just a story.

It looked like I had found a way to avoid dealing with Susan's death and my own feelings, until one day when she received a phone call from her doctor. He explained that the cancer had gone to her leg and she would have to have surgery. When she hung up, I said, "Don't worry, don't worry. This time it's going to be okay. After this surgery, we'll go to this doctor in Mexico. He's curing a lot of people." I began to talk excitedly about this alternative cancer treatment center and she stopped me with a voice I had never heard from her. She screamed at me, "DON'T! Don't say it's going to be okay. It's not going to be okay. What do you know about anything? You've never had one bad thing happen to you. You have this perfect life. You just run around doing things but you're not here for me."

Now at this point in Susan's illness, I had been spending huge amounts of time taking care of her and was shocked to hear her say this. I began to scream back, and we hurled hurtful remarks at each other until all the anger was gone, and only tears were left. I finally said the thing we had been avoiding for more than a year: "I just don't want you to die. If there was only something I could do." And she surprised me totally by saying, "Well, actually there is something you could do. You could make the bed."

I stared at her. She wanted something so simple from me that I couldn't comprehend it. She wanted me to just be with her, to stay still and see her pain and just make her bed because she could no longer do it herself.

As I pulled the comforter back and began to smooth the sheets, I felt more connected to Susan than I ever had and more connected to life. That was the day I began to stop running and doing and accomplishing long enough to see what other people really need. Recently, I amazed myself in how I was able to come through for my mom when she was ill and needed me. And when I stopped running, other people began to come through for me. Somehow I learned how to let the love in. As I support other people, more and more, I experience tremendous support in return . . . from my parents, my friends, my partners, my business associates.

My mother says I have an enchanted life, and she's right, but it's not like it used to be. It's real now. It's deeper and connected to humanity. There's a great deal more love and guardian angels seem to show up regularly.

From Sheila

When I was growing up there were two occupations I had no desire to pursue, perhaps because I was surrounded by both . . . teaching and nursing.

My father, at various points in my school years, was a high school teacher, my elementary school principal, and the superintendent of schools. Whenever my parents entertained friends, the guests were usually teachers. And God forbid if I stepped out of line or played hookey at school, because I had the awesome responsibility of being "the principal's daughter."

My mother was a registered nurse, and though she didn't continue with full-time nursing, she did do private-duty work and taught first aid courses and home health care for the Red Cross. If one of the single teachers (with no family) got sick she was always on hand to help until the teacher got back on his or her feet.

When I began to lead caregiver groups and to work on this book, I began to realize what a powerful legacy had been left to me by each of my parents.

My mother had given me all of my instincts for caregiving. She had taught me many inventive solutions for making things more comfortable and pleasant for someone who is ill—and shown me how the power of a gentle touch and sensitivity came into play in healing the human spirit.

My father had given me his sense of calm, his organization, his need for clarity, and his wry sense of humor. Now, as I see the good this concept is doing, I realize that there are many ways to teach, many ways to nurse, and that you don't have to be a professional to help people.

Being part of Susan's Funny Family put me in touch with those parts of myself that I didn't know were there. Passing the experience on to others is my personal tribute to my parents.

Cappy's Gift

They say that fact is stranger than fiction. In January 2002, eight years after we wrote the first edition of *Share The Care,* Cappy's father was diagnosed with a brain tumor. Just two weeks later, Cappy was also diagnosed with a malignant brain tumor. Ten months later, father and daughter passed from life, a mere twelve hours apart.

It was surreal to form a Share The Care group for her. Her eclectic group of friends and family came together on a cold February evening to unite as Cappy's Brain Trust. The group went beyond those who were in her living room that night; they came from all over the country to help. Over the next ten months things went from bad to worse. Cappy rejected the idea of radiation in favor of an alternative treatment in Texas. Then she left treatment for surgery to reduce the tumor and as a result lost her ability to speak. Back in Houston she lost her ability to walk or even move without assistance. And finally, following emergency surgery, she returned to New York in an alarming condition.

It took over thirty-three of us to keep the life of this one person on track. We helped lift her, we cooked for her, we paid her bills, handled her insurance, and took her to speech therapy, to the movies, and even out to her summerhouse on Long Island. Throughout her ordeal, I was in awe of her courage, strength, and passion. I learned that illness is not necessarily about dying because for her it was all about "how to keep living."

Her Brain Trust grew closer as we worked our way through the weeks and months of emergency rooms visits, hospital stays, and everyday challenges. We came away without realizing that each of us had received a very special gift from Cappy—each other. The superficial acquaintances had become powerful support systems. The person you knew only by name, before the group started, was now someone whose opinion mattered. Now, having lost so much in one person—my co-author, co-worker, and my best friend—I am forever grateful for her "gift of friends."

Her apartment and summerhouse have been sold. Whenever I am in her neighborhood, I look up at her place on the fourteenth floor and see no light or movement. No matter . . . the glow, the enthusiasm, the incredible talent, the bright energy and the special grace and humor that was Cappy lives forever inside the hearts of her family, friends, and all those whose lives she touched.

CHAPTER THIRTY-ONE

A Book with a Mission

From Grass Roots to sharethecaregiving, Inc.

From what we have learned, Share The Care groups have taken hold mostly by word of mouth. Usually an individual who has been part of a group will make efforts to let others in their community or church know about the model and what a valuable tool it has been to help other individuals or families struggling to be caregivers and make a living. Part of the dream is to have sharethecaregiving centers around the country where people can find information and support from others in the area who have been through this experience. In Marshfield, Wisconsin, a former group participant named Mindy has started a Share The Care Station designed to do just that within a community coalition.

The word has even been spread by care recipients, as in the case of Michelle, the subject of a video produced by the University of Wisconsin's Comprehensive Cancer Center (UWCCC). Claire Culbertson, Director of Outreach and Volunteers for sharethecaregiving, said that Michelle not only allowed the video camera into her life but she was often a speaker at the UWCCC presentations on Share The Care to caregivers and health professionals. We have lost Michelle, but her beauty and grace under the most difficult circumstances will be forever remembered through the compassionate video about her wonderful group.

Besides helping friends or neighbors who have little or no family or whose family lives far away, Share The Care has come to the rescue of many families when a spouse has been diagnosed with a serious illness. This is how Amrita describes her circumstance.

> The main thing I want to share is how this group seems to be evolving for a family unit. We are in a relatively rare (but still too common) position of dealing with end of life and beginning of life simultaneously. What to do when there is a stay-at-home mom, with two young children (mine are two and six), and the breadwinner gets sick? The group helps with meals and child care, which enables me to be more available to assist my husband and work on the medical/healing aspects. They also help me in transitioning into taking over in all the (shockingly traditional) roles he was handling in our family enterprise; for example, house repairs, car maintenance, home maintenance, computers and other technology, and finances, as well as bringing in money. I would be completely overwhelmed without our Share The Care Sangha group.

Groups come in all shapes and sizes, from a handful of people to as many as a hundred volunteers. Peg's Legs, one such very large group, recently contacted me from Honolulu, Hawaii. Some people in groups are even chronically ill themselves, yet intent on helping others. Pat told us what she got from being in a Share The Care group even though she was coping with her own health issues at the same time:

> The feeling that my life was still important, I am not just someone with fibromyalgia. I have things to give; sometimes this is difficult for me to remember because I am in pain at some level 24/7 since July 1988. I sometimes need to be reminded that I am still a worthwhile person.

People who use the Share The Care model can learn to become better collaborators when it comes to teamwork or other group involvements. And they come out the other side richer for the experience, stronger as people, better able to cope with what life hands them, and feeling good about themselves. As Mary put it:

> I can't begin to describe how proud I am to have been part of this. It was the most enriching experience ever. An incredible learning of what is in-

volved in being a caretaker and how such a group can truly help. I was fascinated by the process: the incredible volunteership that would come through, the emotional roller-coaster ride, how complete strangers would reveal little parts of themselves by e-mail, and actually how much love went between members of the group.

Group and family members have voiced the great value in making this model widely known to others. Kathryn, the wife of a care recipient, said about *Share The Care:*

I think the book was the best piece of information we received in all our searching. It is the greatest and I recommend it to everyone who asks about our situation. I wish that all hospitals could hand it out when they give you a diagnosis for ALS. I wish you could get a grant to have it placed in every hospital waiting room and doctor's office. Everyone knows someone that could benefit from reading it.

sharethecaregiving, Inc. — *The Road Ahead*

March 1, 2004

In 2003, to honor the memory of my late co-author and best friend, Cappy Capossela, I founded sharethecaregiving, Inc. The organization has filed its application for recognition for exemption with the Internal Revenue Service and has registered with the Charities Bureau of the New York State Department of Law. We hope to have IRS confirmation of our 501(c)3 status very soon.

The mission of sharethecaregiving is to promote group caregiving as a proven option for meeting the needs of the seriously ill, chronically ill, those in rehabilitation, or the elderly and their caregivers. The organization will seek to reach, inform, and educate struggling caregivers, as well as health-care professionals, communities, clergy, and corporations, about the Share The Care model.

One of the biggest challenges for sharethecaregiving will be to locate and learn about all the Share The Care groups that have been formed, are currently at work, or are planned for the near future. If you have been, or currently are, part of a group, and have seen and experienced a real difference in the quality of life for your friend or family member, we would love to know about it.

On the Web site, http://www.sharethecare.org, we have created a questionnaire (click on the JOIN US button), and we invite you to send us your information. Any feedback we collect will only be used to help and to teach other groups and to make improvements in the Share The Care system. If you would like to submit a story and pictures about your group for consideration on the Share The Care Web site, please click on the YOUR STORIES button for more information.

To learn about the most current information and developments with the sharethecaregiving organization, please check the Web site. Your questions and comments are most welcome. You can e-mail or write us at:

sharethecaregiving, Inc.
320 East 35th Street, Suite 3B
New York, NY 10016

sharethecaregiving offers lectures, seminars, and workshops. If you would like to more information, please call or e-mail:
sw_npo@sharethecare.org
Tel: 212-686-9254
Web site: http://www.sharethecare.org

ဢ

A copy of our latest annual report can be obtained by writing to the Attorney General, Department of Law, Charities Bureau, 120 Broadway, New York, NY 10271, or by contacting sharethecare giving, Inc.

Share The Care book rights are owned by sharethecaregiving, Inc.

Bibliographic Resources

HELPFUL BOOKS

Note: While only printed material is included here, many of these books are also available as audiocassettes and/or CDs.

After Death: Mapping the Journey. Sukie Miller and Suzanne Lipsett. New York: Simon & Schuster, 1997.

After Mastectomy: Healing Physically and Emotionally. Rosalind Benedet. Omaha, NE: Addicus, 2003.

Alzheimer's Activities: Hundreds of Activities for Men and Women with Alzheimer's Disease and Related Disorders. B. J. FitzRay. Windsor, CA: Rayve Productions, 2001.

The Caregiver's Book: Caring for Another, Caring for Yourself. James Miller. Minneapolis: Augsburg Fortress, 1996.

The Caregiver's Essential Handbook: More Than 1,200 Tips to Help You Care for and Comfort the Seniors in Your Life. Sasha Carr and Sandra Choron. New York: McGraw-Hill, 2003.

Caregiving: The Spiritual Journey of Love, Loss, and Renewal. Beth Witrogen McLeod. Hoboken, NJ: Wiley, 1999.

Caring for the Patient with Cancer at Home: A Guide for Patients and Families. American Cancer Society. Rev. ed. 2003. Available online or call the ACS (1-800-227-2345). http://www.cancer.org/docroot/MBC/content/MBC_2_3x_Caring_for_the_Patient_with_Cancer_at_Home_A_Guide_for_Patients_and_Families.asp (accessed April 20, 2004).

Caring for Yourself While Caring for Your Aging Parents: How to Help, How to Survive, 2nd ed. Claire Berman. New York: Holt/Owl Books, 2001.

Choices in Healing: Integrating the Best of Conventional and Complementary Approaches to Cancer. Michael Lerner. Cambridge, MA: MIT, 1996. Available online. http://www.commonweal.org/choicescontents.html (accessed April 20, 2004).

The Complete Bedside Companion: No-Nonsense Advice on Caring for the Seriously Ill. Rodger McFarlane and Philip Bashe. New York: Simon & Schuster, 1998.

Death: The Final Stage of Growth. Elisabeth Kübler-Ross, ed. Englewood Cliffs, NJ: Prentice-Hall, 1975. Pb. reprint, New York: Simon & Schuster/Touchstone, 1986. Pb. reprint, New York: Scribner, 1997.

Diagnosis: Cancer: Your Guide to the First Months of Healthy Survivorship, 3rd ed. Wendy Schlessel Harpham. New York: Norton, 2003.

Dr. Susan Love's Breast Book, 3rd ed. Susan M. Love with Karen Lindsey. New York: Perseus, 2000.

Elder Rage, or Take My Father . . . Please!: How to Survive Caring for Aging Parents. Jacqueline Marcell. Irvine, CA: Impressive Press, 2001.

Facing Death and Finding Hope: A Guide to the Emotional and Spiritual Care of the Dying. Christine Longaker. New York: Doubleday, 1997. Pb. reprint, New York: Doubleday/Main Street, 1998.

The Fearless Caregiver: How to Get the Best Care for Your Loved One and Still Have a Life of Your Own. Gary Barg, ed. Sterling, VA: Capital, 2001. Pb. reprint, Sterling, VA: Capital, 2003.

Finding Hope When a Child Dies: What Other Cultures Can Teach Us. Sukie Miller with Doris Ober. New York: Simon & Schuster, 1999.

Healing: A Guide to Recovery After Lumpectomy. Rosalind Benedet. San Francisco: Benedet, 1996.

Healing: A Guide to Recovery After Mastectomy. Rosalind Benedet. San Francisco: Benedet, 1996.

Healing into Life and Death. Stephen Levine. Garden City, NY: Doubleday/Anchor, 1987.

The Heart of Healing: Companion to the TBS Television Series The Heart of Healing. Institute of Noetic Sciences with William Poole. Atlanta: Turner, 1993.

Helping Yourself Help Others: A Book for Caregivers. Rosalynn Carter with Susan K. Golant. New York: Times Books, 1994. Pb. reprint, New York: Three Rivers Press, 1995.

How to Care for Aging Parents. Virginia Morris. New York: Workman, 1996.

How to Survive the Loss of a Love: 58 Things to Do When There Is Nothing to Be Done. Melba Colgrove, Harold Bloomfield, and Peter McWilliams. New York: Leo Press (Simon & Schuster, dist.), 1976. Pb. reprint, New York: Bantam, 1982. Large print ed., New York: G. K. Hall, 1992. 3rd ed., Los Angeles: Prelude Press, 1993.

It's Always Something. Gilda Radner. New York: Simon & Schuster, 1989. Pb. reprint, New York: Avon, 2000.

Kitchen Table Wisdom: Stories That Heal. Rachel Naomi Remen. New York: Riverhead, 1996. Pb. reprint, New York: Riverhead, 1997.

Learning to Fall: The Blessings of an Imperfect Life. Phillip Simmons. New York: Bantam, 2002.

Learning to Speak Alzheimer's: A Groundbreaking Approach for Everyone Dealing with the Disease. Joanne Koenig Coste. Boston: Houghton Mifflin, 2003.

Living in the Light: A Guide to Personal and Planetary Transformation. Shakti Gawain with Laurel King. Novato, CA: Whatever Publishing, 1986. Pb. reprint, New York: Bantam, 1993. Rev. ed., Novato, CA: New World, 1998.

Love, Honor, and Value. Suzanne Geffen Mintz. Sterling, VA: Capital Books, 2002.

Making Life More Livable: A Practical Guide to Over 1,000 Products and Resources for Living in the Mature Years. Ellen Lederman. New York: Simon & Schuster/Fireside, 1994.

Questions and Answers on Death and Dying: A Companion Volume to On Death and Dying. Elisabeth Kübler-Ross. New York: Macmillan/Collier, 1974. Pb. reprint, New York: Scribner, 1997. Pb. reprint, New York: Simon & Schuster/ Touchstone, 1997.

Start the Conversation: The Book About Death You Were Hoping to Find. Ganga Stone. New York: Warner, 1996.

The Tibetan Book of Living and Dying. Sogyal Rinpoche. San Francisco: HarperSanFrancisco, 1992. Rev. ed., San Francisco: HarperSanFrancisco, 2002.

To Live Until We Say Good-Bye. Elisabeth Kübler-Ross. New York: Simon & Schuster/Fireside, 1978. Pb. reprint, New York: Scribners, 1997.

Understanding Lumpectomy: A Treatment Guide for Breast Cancer. Rosalind Benedet and Mark C. Rounsaville. Omaha, NE: Addicus, 2004.

When Life Becomes Precious: The Essential Guide for Patients, Loved Ones, and Friends of Those Facing Serious Illnesses. Elise NeeDell Babcock. New York: Bantam, 1997.

When Your Friend Gets Cancer: How You Can Help. Amy Harwell with Kristine Tomasik. Wheaton, IL: Harold Shaw, 1987.

You Can Heal Your Life. Louise L. Hay. Carlsbad, CA: Hay House, 1984.

SPECIAL INTEREST BOOKS

Altars: Bringing Sacred Shrines into Your Everyday Life. Denise Linn. New York: Wellspring/Ballantine, 1999.

Clear Your Clutter with Feng Shui. Karen Kingston. New York: Broadway Books, 1999.

Colour Scents: Healing with Colour and Aroma. Suzy Chiazzari. Essex, UK: C.W. Daniel, 1998.

The Complete Book of Essential Oils and Aromatherapy. Valerie Ann Worwood. Novato, CA: New World, 1991.

Creative Visualization: Use the Power of Your Imagination to Create What You Want in Your Life. Shakti Gawain. Novato, CA: Whatever Publishing, 1978. Pb. reprint, New York: Bantam, 1983. 3rd ed., Novato, CA: New World, 1998.

Feng Shui and Health: The Anatomy of a Home: Using Feng Shui to Disarm Illness, Accelerate Recovery, and Create Optimal Health. Nancy SantoPietro. New York: Three Rivers, 2002.

Organizing from the Inside Out. Julie Morgenstern. New York: Holt/Owl Books, 1998.

HELPFUL NEWSLETTERS AND MAGAZINES

Eldercare911. Subscribe to this monthly electronic newsletter online: http://www .eldercare911handbook.com/newsletter.html

Take Care! Self Care for the Family Caregiver. This quarterly newsletter is a benefit of membership in the National Family Caregivers Association. Membership is free to family caregivers in the United States. Join online at http://www .nfcacares.org/ or call 1-800-896-3650.

Today's Caregiver. Caregivers can request a free online newsletter or purchase a subscription to the print magazine at http://www.caregiver.com/. The Web site also offers back issues of articles from *Today's Caregiver.*

Helpful Associations

AGING

Aging With Dignity
40960 California Oaks Road #221
Murrieta, CA 92562
909-696-0378
http://www.agingwithdignity.com

Alliance for Aging Research
2021 K Street NW, Suite 305
Washington, DC 20006
202-293-2856
http://www.agingresearch.org

American Association of Homes and Services for the Aging (AAHSA)
2519 Connecticut Avenue NW
Washington, DC 20008
202-783-2242
http://www.aahsa.org

American Association of Retired Persons (AARP)
601 E Street NW
Washington, DC 20049
800-424-3410; 888-OUR-AARP (888-687-2277)
http://www.aarp.org

Children of Aging Parents
1609 Woodbourne Road, Suite 302-A
Levittown, PA 19057
215-945-6900; 800-227-7294
http://www.caps4caregivers.org

ElderCare Online
50 Amuxen Court
Islip, NY 11751
http://www.ec-online.net

ElderHope
ElderHope, LLC
PO Box 940822
Plano, TX 75094
972-768-8553
http://www.elderhope.com

Medicare Rights Center
1460 Broadway, 17th floor
New York, NY 10036
212-869-3850
http://www.medicarerights.org

National Association for Continence (NAFC)
PO Box 1019
Charleston, SC 29402

800-BLADDER (800-252-3337);
843-377-0900
http://www.nafc.org

**National Council on the Aging
(NCOA)**
300 D Street SW, Suite 801
Washington, DC 20024
202-479-1200
http://www.ncoa.org

AIDS

Gay Men's Health Crisis (GMHC)
The Tisch Building
119 West 24th Street
New York, NY 10011
212-367-1000
http://www.gmhc.org

GMHC hotline
212-807-6655 or 800-AIDS-NYC or
hotline@gmhc.org

Project Inform
205 13th Street, Suite 2001
San Francisco, CA 94103
415-558-8669
Treatment hotline: 800-822-7422 or
415-558-9051
http://www.projectinform.org

ALS

**The ALS Association (Amyotrophic
Lateral Sclerosis Association)**
27001 Agoura Road, Suite 150
Calabasas Hills, CA 91301
Information/referral service: 800-
782-4747
All others: 818-880-9007
http://www.alsa.org

ALZHEIMER'S

Alzheimer's Association
225 North Michigan Avenue,
Suite 1700
Chicago, IL 60601
800-272-3900; 312-335-8700
http://www.alz.org

BLINDNESS

**American Foundation for the Blind
(AFB)**
11 Penn Plaza, Suite 300
New York, NY 10001
212-502-7600; 800-AFB-LINE (800-
232-5463)
http://www.afb.org

**National Association for Visually
Handicapped**
22 West 21st Street, 6th floor
New York, NY 10010
212-889-3141

3201 Balboa Street
San Francisco, CA 94121
415-221-3201
http://www.navh.org

CANCER (See also *Research*)

**American Brain Tumor Association
(ABTA)**
2720 River Road
Des Plaines, IL 60018
847-827-9910
Patient line: 800-886-2282
http://www.abta.org

American Cancer Society
1599 Clifton Road NE

Atlanta, GA 30329
800-ACS-2345 (800-227-2345)
http://www.cancer.org

Cancer and Careers
Cosmetic Executive Women
21 East 40th Street, Suite 1700
New York, NY 10016
http://www.cancerandcareers.org

Cancer Care
275 Seventh Avenue
New York, NY 10001
800-813-4673
http://www.cancercare.org

Cancer Shock
http://www.cancershock.com

Colon Cancer Alliance
175 Ninth Avenue
New York, NY 10011
877-422-2030
http://www.ccalliance.org

Gillette Women's Cancer Connection
http://www.gillettecancerconnect.org

Kidney Cancer Association
1234 Sherman Avenue, Suite 203
Evanston, IL 60202
847-332-1051, 800-850-9132
www.kidneycancerassociation.org

Leukemia & Lymphoma Society
1311 Mamaroneck Avenue
White Plains, NY 10605
914-949-5213
http://www.leukemia-lymphoma.org

National Brain Tumor Foundation
414 13th Street, Suite 700

Oakland, CA 94612
510-839-9777; 800-934-CURE
(800-934-2873)
http://www.braintumor.org

National Ovarian Cancer Coalition (NOCC)
500 NE Spanish River Boulevard,
Suite 8
Boca Raton, FL 33431
561-393-0005
888-OVARIAN (888-682-7426)
http://www.ovarian.org

Susan G. Komen Breast Cancer Foundation
5005 LBJ Freeway, Suite 250
Dallas, TX 75244
972-855-1600
800-I'M-AWARE
(800-462-9273)
http://www.komen.org

University of Wisconsin Comprehensive Cancer Center
600 Highland Avenue K5/601
Madison, WI 53792
608-263-8600
http://www.cancer.wisc.edu/services/
frameservices.html

USTOO! International, Inc. (Prostate Cancer)
5003 Fairview Avenue
Downers Grove, IL 60515
630-795-1002
800-80-USTOO (800-808-7866)
http://www.ustoo.com

Washingtonian Online (Breast Cancer Help)
www.washingtonian.com/health/
breast_cancer_help.html

Women's Cancer Network (WCN)
230 West Monroe, Suite 2528
Chicago, IL 60606
312-578-1439
http://www.wcn.org

Y-ME National Breast Cancer Organization
212 West Van Buren, Suite 1000
Chicago, IL 60697
312-986-8338
800-221-2141 (English); 800-986-9505 (Español)
http://www.y-me.org

CANCER RESOURCES FOR TEENS AND CHILDREN

Brave Kids
1510 11th Street, Suite 203
Santa Monica, CA 90401
800-568-1008
http://www.bravekids.org

Candlelighters Childhood Cancer Foundation
PO Box 498
Kensington, MD 20895
301-962-3520
800-366-CCCF (800-366-2223)
http://www.candlelighters.org

Children's Hospice International
See under *Hospice*

Kids Konnected
27071 Cabot Road, Suite 102
Laguna Hills, CA 92653
949-582-5443
http://www.kidskonnected.org

Planet Cancer
3710 Cedar Street, Box 11

Austin, TX 78705
512-452-9010
http://www.planetcancer.org

TLC—Teens Living with Cancer
Melissa's Living Legacy Foundation
245 Citation Drive
Henrietta, NY 14467
585-334-0858
http://www.teenslivingwithcancer.org

CAREGIVING

Family Caregiver Alliance
690 Market Street, Suite 600
San Francisco, CA 94104
415-434-3388
800-445-8106
http://www.caregiver.org

Gilda's Club Worldwide
322 Eighth Avenue, Suite 1402
New York, NY 10001
888-GILDA-4-U (888-445-3248)
http://www.Gildasclub.org

National Alliance for Caregiving
4720 Montgomery Lane, 5th Floor
Bethesda, MD 20814
http://www.caregiving.org

National Family Caregivers Association
10400 Connecticut Avenue, #500
Kensington, MD 26895
800-896-3650
http://www.nfcacares.org

National Organization For Empowering Caregivers (NOFEC)
http://www.nofec.org
Empowering Caregivers
http://www.care-givers.com

425 West 23rd Street, Suite 9B
New York, NY 10011
212-807-1204

Patient Advocate Foundation (PAF)
700 Thimble Shoals Blvd., Suite 200
Newport News, VA 23606
800-532-5274
http://www.patientadvocate.org

COMMUNICATIONS

CaringBridge—a nonprofit service
that offers free Web pages for friends
and family of patients undergoing
treatment, rehabilitation, or end-of-
life care
4607 Beacon Hill, Suite 200
Eagan, MN 55122
651-452-7940
http://www.caringbridge.org

DIABETES

American Diabetes Association
National Call Center
1701 North Beauregard Street
Alexandria, VA 22311
800-DIABETES (800-342-2383)
http://www.diabetes.org

END-OF-LIFE ISSUES AND ADVANCE DIRECTIVES

Aging with Dignity—Five Wishes
PO Box 1661
Tallahassee, FL 32302
850-681-2010
http://www.agingwithdignity.org/
Aging with Dignity offers for sale for a
nominal fee the "Five Wishes"
document developed in conjunction
with the American Bar Association to

help plan end-of-life issues on the
medical, personal, emotional, and
spiritual levels.

Dying Well
http://www.dyingwell.org

The Funeral Directory
http://www.thefuneraldirectory.com
Arranging, pre-planning,
bereavement, critical care, eldercare.

Last Acts
http://www.lastacts.org
Last Acts has joined Partnership for
Caring to form Last Acts Partnership.
These and many other organizations
have joined to urge an improvement
in end-of-life care and caring. The
Web site offers a wide variety of
resources.

Partnership for Caring
1620 Eye Street NW, Suite 212
Washington, DC 20006
202-296-8071
800-989-9455
http://www.partnershipforcaring.org
Last Acts Partnership provides
information on Advance Directives
and other end-of-life issues.
The Web site also offers free down-
loadable medical power of attorney
documents and state-specific living
wills.

Webdirectives
PO Box 1855
Dunedin, FL 34697
866-304-4674
727-423-8466
http://www.webdirectives.com
For a fee, this company stores health-

care and medical-direction documents online.

EQUIPMENT/SUPPLIES/RAMPS

Caregiver Marketplace
The Caregivers Group, Inc.
PO Box 1206
Charlestown, RI 02813
401-364-9100
http://www.caregiversmarket
place.com
This site sells a wide variety of health-care products and equipment with discount and cash-back options.

LifeFone
1-800-882-2280
http://www.lifeFone.com
Monitors and personal emergency response systems.

Medic Alert Foundation International
888-633-4298
http://www.medicalert.org
Medical ID and emergency response center.

Resources for Disabled Online
http://www.spinalcord.uab.edu
University of Alabama (Department of Rehabilitation Medicine) has compiled links to extensive resources—equipment and accessibility applicable to many illnesses and disabilities.

The SunBox Company
19217 Orbit Drive
Gaithersburg, MD 20879
800-548-3968

http://www.sunbox.com
One of many firms offering special lamps for light therapy.

HEART DISEASE

American Heart Association
7272 Greenville Avenue
Dallas, TX 75231
800-AHA-USA-1 (800-242-8721)
http://www.americanheart.org

Mended Hearts, Inc.
7272 Greenville Avenue
Dallas, TX 75231
214-706-1442
http://www.mendedhearts.org

HOSPICE

American Hospice Foundation
2120 L Street NW, Suite 200
Washington, DC 20037
202-223-0204
http://www.americanhospice.org

Childrens Hospice International
901 North Pitt Street, Suite 230
Alexandria, VA 22314
703-684-0330
800-2-4-CHILD (800-242-4453)
http://www.chionline.org

Hospice Education Institute
3 Unity Square, PO Box 98
Machiasport, ME 04655
207-255-8800
800-331-1620
http://www.hospiceworld.org

Hospice Foundation of America
2001 S Street NW, #300
Washington, DC 20009

800-854-3402
http://www.hospicefoundation.org

Hospice web
http://www.hospiceweb.com

National Hospice and Palliative Care Organization (NHPCO)
1700 Diagonal Road, Suite 625
Alexandria, VA 22314
703-837-1500
http://www.nhpco.org

KIDNEY DISEASE

American Kidney Fund (AKF)
6110 Executive Boulevard,
Suite 1010
Rockville, MD 20852
800-638-8299
http://www.akfinc.org

Kidney Cancer Association
1234 Sherman Avenue, Suite 203
Evanston, IL 60202
847-332-1051; 800-850-9132
http://www.kidneycancerassociation
.org

Kidney Transplant/Dialysis Association, Inc.
PO Box 51362 GMF
Boston, MA 02205-1362
781-641-4000 (voice mail)
http://www.ktda.org

National Kidney Foundation
30 East 33rd Street, Suite 1100
New York, NY 10016
212-889-2210
800-622-9010
http://www.kidney.org

LIVER

American Liver Foundation
75 Maiden Lane, Suite 603
New York, NY 10038
212-668-1000
800-GO-LIVER (800-465-4837)
888-4HEP.USA (888-443-7872)
http://www.liverfoundation.org

LUNG DISEASE

American Lung Association
61 Broadway, 6th floor
New York, NY 10006
212-315-8700
800-LUNG-USA (800-586-4872)
800-548-8252
http://www.lungusa.org

MULTIPLE SCLEROSIS

National Multiple Sclerosis Society
733 Third Avenue
New York, NY 10019
800-FIGHT-MS (800-344-4867)
http://www.nationalmssociety.org

MUSCULAR DYSTROPHY

Muscular Dystrophy Association
3300 E. Sunrise Drive
Tucson, AZ 85718
800-572-1717
http://www.mdausa.org

ORGAN DONATION

The Living Bank
PO Box 6725
Houston, TX 77265
800-528-2971
http://www.livingbank.org

PAIN

New York Online Access to Health (NOAH)
http://www.noah-health.org
Full-text access to consumer health information in English and Spanish.

Pain
http://www.pain.com
"A world of information on pain" and how to deal with it.

PARALYSIS

Christopher Reeve Paralysis Foundation
500 Morris Avenue
Springfield, NJ 07081
800-225-0292
800-539-7309
http://www.paralysis.org

Paralyzed Veterans of America (PVA)
801 18th Street NW
Washington, DC 20006
800-424-8200
Hotline: 800-232-1782
http://www.pva.org

Spinal Cord Injury Information Network
http://www.spinalcord.uab.edu

PARKINSON'S DISEASE

American Parkinson Disease Association, Inc.
1250 Hylan Blvd., Suite 4B
Staten Island, NY 10301
718-981-8001
800-223-2732
10850 Wilshire Blvd., Suite 730
Los Angeles, CA 90024
800-908-2732
310-474-5391
http://www.apdaparkinson.org

RESEARCH

About Cancer
http://www.cancer.about.com
Extensive collection of links and articles.

Cancer Decisions (The Moss Reports)
PO Box 1076
Lemont, PA 16851
800-980-1234
http://www.cancerdecisions.com
Information and referral service offering in-depth information on specific cancers.

Cancer Yellow Pages
PO Box 21501
Tampa, FL 33622
http://www.canceryellowpages.com
Directory of U.S. doctors who treat cancer patients.

HealthFinder
PO Box 1133
Washington, DC 20013
http://www.healthfinder.gov
U.S. Dept. of Health and Human Services site.

National Library of Medicine
http://www.nlm.nih.gov
Medline service of the National Library of Medicine and National Institutes of Health.

STROKE

American Stroke Association
7272 Greenville Avenue
Dallas, TX 75231
888-4-STROKE (888-478-7653)
http://www.strokeassociation.org

National Institute of Neurological Disorders and Stroke (NINDS)
NIH Neurological Institute
PO Box 5801
Bethesda, MD 20824
301-496-5751
800-352-9424
http://www.ninds.nih.gov

National Stroke Association
9707 E. Easter Lane
Englewood, CO 80112
800-STROKES (800-787-6537)
http://www.stroke.org

TRANSPORTATION AND HOUSING

American Cancer Society
1599 Clifton Road NE
Atlanta, GA 30329
800-ACS-2345 (800-227-2345)
http://www.cancer.org
Search the site for "Hope Lodge." This program arranges free hotel/motel accommodations for cancer patients receiving treatment far from home and sometimes also for their caregiver.

Angel Flight Northeast
Lawrence Municipal Airport
492 Sutton Street
North Andover, MA 01845

800-549-9980 for flight requests
Office: 978-794-6868
http://www.angelflightne.org
Volunteer pilots provide free air transportation in private aircraft for patients who need to travel for life-saving medical care.

Corporate Angel Network, Inc.
Westchester County Airport
One Loop Road
White Plains, NY 10604
914-328-1313
http://www.corpangelnetwork.org
CAN arranges free air transportation in the empty seats of corporate jets for cancer patients traveling to approved medical facilities.

National Association of Hospital Hospitality Houses, Inc.
Mailing address:
PO Box 18087
Asheville, NC 28814
Physical address:
44 Merrimon Avenue, 1st Floor
Asheville, NC 28801
828-253-1188
800-542-9730
828-253-8082
http://www.nahhh.org
NAHHH is an association of more than 150 nonprofit organizations located throughout the United States that provide family-centered lodging and support services to families and their loved ones who are receiving medical treatment far from their home communities.

Ronald McDonald House Charities— low-cost temporary housing for families of seriously ill children.

One Kroc Drive
Oak Brook, IL 60523
630-623-7048
http://www.rmhc.com
This contact information is basically
for national and international
administrative business. To request

low-cost temporary housing for the
family of a seriously ill child who is
being treated in a hospital far from
home, contact a local Ronald
McDonald house. A search tool on
the Web site will help you locate the
nearest one.

Index